PARENTING TEENS WITH ADHD

The Ultimate Handbook for Parents to support their Child with ADHD to Improve Focus, Organization, Motivation and Handle Emotions with Confidence and Success

Kai M. Jordan

SWENETT

To all the parents navigating the unique challenges and joys of raising teenagers with ADHD. Your unwavering love, patience, and dedication inspire hope and strength. This book is dedicated to you, for your tireless commitment to supporting your children as they navigate the complexities of adolescence with courage and resilience.

In the journey of parenting, every obstacle becomes an opportunity for growth, every challenge a chance to learn, and every moment of frustration a reminder of the boundless love that fuels our dedication.

UNKNOWN

CONTENTS

Title Page

Copyright

Dedication

Epigraph

Introduction

Preface

Your Free Gift 1

Part 1: I Have ADHD, Now What? 5

Chapter 1: The Truth About ADHD 6

Part 2: Schooling With ADHD 21

Chapter 2: Executive Functioning and ADHD 22

Chapter 3: Discover Your Strengths and Understand Your Weaknesses 33

Chapter 4: Get Organized 43

Chapter 5: Know Your Study Style 55

Chapter 6: Utilize the Power of Color Coding 65

Chapter 7: Write, Write, Write! 74

Chapter 8: Setting Goals 84

Chapter 9: Utilize Phone Apps 97

Chapter 10: Stay Motivated 106
Part 3: Home and Life With ADHD 116
Chapter 11: Managing Emotional Development/ Understand Your Emotions 117
Chapter 12: Utilize Hyperfocus 129
Chapter 13: Your Teens Activities 139
Chapter 14: Social Development/Interacting With Others 151
Chapter 15: Self-Esteem 163
Chapter 16: Know Yourself Better, Build Your Confidence, and Believe in Yourself 173
Conclusion 182
Thank You 187
References 188
About The Author 193
Focus Forward: Navigating ADHD 195
Books By This Author 201

INTRODUCTION

ADHD isn't a bad thing; it's a different way of thinking. –
David Neeleman

Aisha marched across the stage to thunderous applause. She took her diploma with a firm handshake and turned to beam at her mother, Paige, who was sitting in the front row.

"You did it, baby girl!" Aisha's mother roared over the sound of her classmates cheering. Watching her daughter graduate was the most rewarding moment of Paige's entire life. You see, three years ago, Aisha was failing every subject. In fact, Paige's school attendance was so poor that she faced serious reprimands.

Aisha was diagnosed with ADHD when she was ten years old, and it only escalated from that point on. No matter what they tried, Aisha just couldn't seem to overcome her explosive behaviour, disorganization, and hyperactivity.

It was only when Paige came to understand that there was nothing *wrong* with her child but that she was simply *different* that they began to realize that this could be with her time management, organization, prioritizing, and negative thinking.

It wasn't easy, but under Paige's loving guidance, Aisha was able to learn new coping mechanisms that boosted her confidence and self-esteem. Soon, she was able to work on her social skills and emotional regulation; her aggressive outbursts became few and far between, and her attendance at school improved dramatically. As she discovered new time management and organization skills, her grades also began to improve.

The culmination of all their hard work was that Aisha was now graduating and had been offered a scholarship to Michigan, where she was joining the volleyball team. Her life was completely transformed.

If you are the parent of a teenager with ADHD, you have probably endured years of phone calls from exasperated teachers, watched your child struggle to keep friends, and stayed up late agonizing over how to help them survive and thrive in this world, just as Paige did. Parenting a teen with ADHD can be unrelentingly hard.

But there is hope. In this book, I will draw on the latest scientific research and my over 15 years of experience coaching families impacted by ADHD to provide a practical system to help your teen succeed in school, at home, and in relationships.

PREFACE

Parenting is a journey filled with twists and turns, challenges and triumphs. When your child has ADHD, this journey can often feel like navigating uncharted waters in a storm. As a life coach dealing with many parents and teenagers with ADHD, I understand the unique struggles, frustrations, and joys that come with this territory.

In writing this book, my goal is simple: to offer support, guidance, and reassurance to parents who are raising teens with ADHD. Drawing upon my own experiences, as well as insights from experts in the field, I aim to provide practical strategies and heartfelt encouragement for navigating the teenage years with grace and resilience.

This book is not a one-size-fits-all solution, nor is it a roadmap with all the answers. Instead, think of it as a companion on your journey - a source of comfort and inspiration as you navigate the highs and lows of parenting a teenager with ADHD. Together, let us embrace the challenges, celebrate the victories, and cherish the journey ahead.

With warmth and empathy,

Kai

YOUR FREE GIFT

As a way of saying thanks for your purchase, I'm offering ***The ADHD Relationship Evaluation and Money Management Worksheet*** for FREE to my readers.

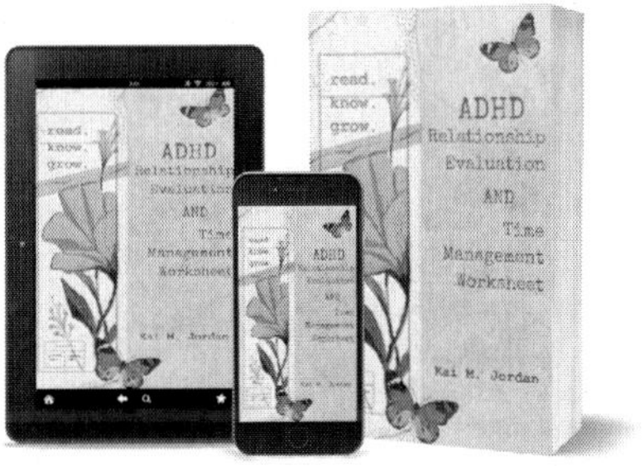

Plus, you will get ***The Decluttering and Organizing Bundle*** for FREE .

This valuable package includes four valuable components:

1. The Decluttering Booklet (42 decluttering exercises + 22 self-reflection pages + inspirational quotes).

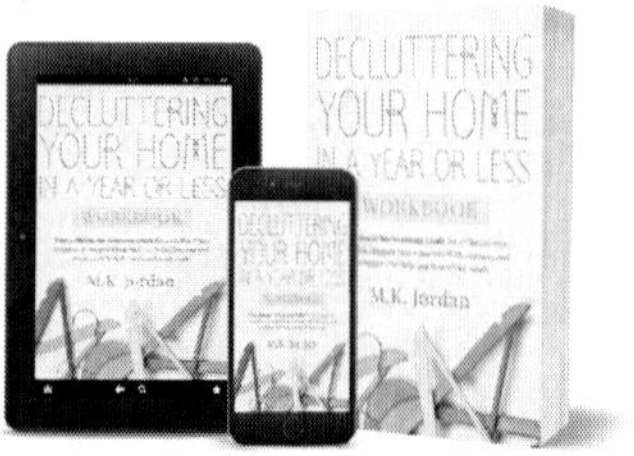

2. The Decluttering Journal & Planner (30-steps to Declutter your home).

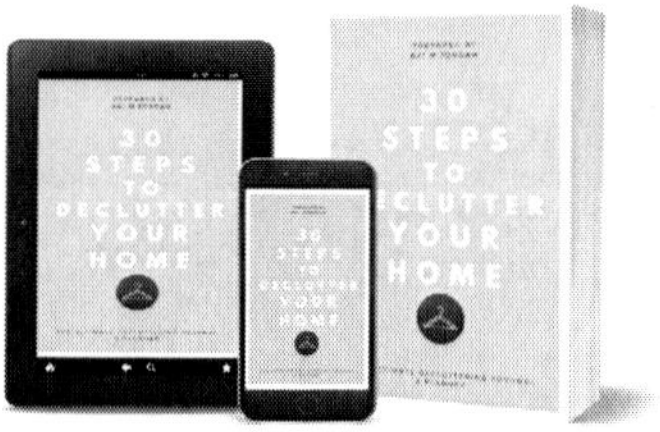

3. The Ultimate Decluttering Checklist

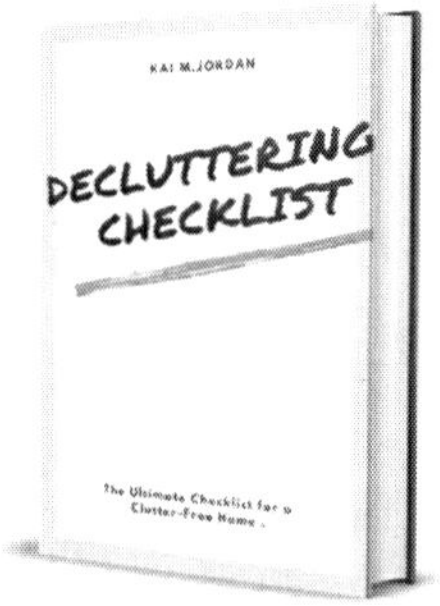

4. Let Go of Clutter: Supply Checklist, and Stay the Course Worksheet

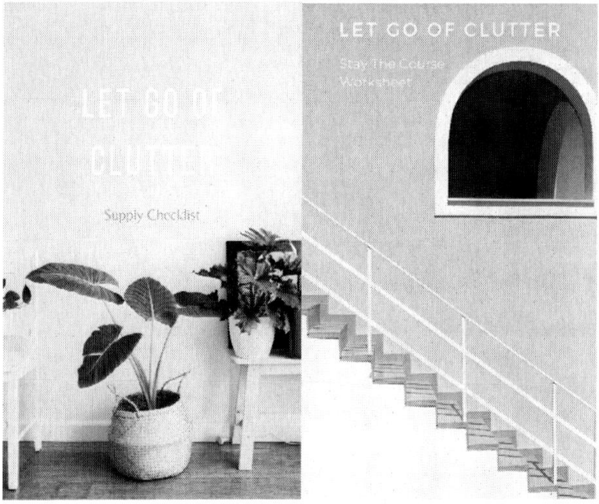

To get instant access just go to:

http://swenettbooks.com

or Just Scan this Code by Your Phone

Inside the bundle, you will get:

- 42 practical decluttering exercises in the book in a printable coloured nice format.
- 22 self-reflection pages in the book in a printable coloured format.
- 262 pages of Decluttering Journal in a bright watercolour design.
- Perfect 30-step plan for Decluttering your home.
- Ultimate Checklist for Decluttering which will save you hours of your decluttering time and skyrocket your productivity

- Let Go of Clutter: supply checklist.
- Stay The Course Worksheet.

If you want to get the maximum benefit through your organizing your home journey, make sure to grab the free bundle **NOW**!

PART 1: I HAVE ADHD, NOW WHAT?

CHAPTER 1: THE TRUTH ABOUT ADHD

We're living in a time where neurodivergence is more broadly understood or even accepted – with people learning about the ways conditions like Autism and ADHD have historically been underdiagnosed or underreported, especially in women. –Holly Smale

Tairae reached up and grabbed his father's free hand as they walked out of the neurology office. Aiden looked down at his son's dark hair and then looked at the bundle of ADHD paperwork in his other hand.

All those teacher phone calls, Tairae's disaster bedroom, and the epic meltdowns all suddenly made sense. ADHD. There was a deeper meaning behind it all, after all.

The doctor had explained it all to them kindly, saying that Tairae's brain just operated differently. He wasn't broken or damaged, and he would thrive with the right guidance tailored to his unique mind.

Aiden smiled up at his father nervously, too young to really understand everything that had just been told but old enough to know that this was a really important day for them as a family.

"We've got this, kiddo," Aiden told him warmly.

What Is ADHD?

ADHD is a common neurodevelopmental disorder that typically appears in childhood and is characterized by difficulty paying attention, excessive activity, and trouble controlling impulsive behaviour (CDC, 2023).

ADHD was first formally recognized as a mental disorder in the 1960s (Holland, 2021). Before that time, the symptoms were often viewed as simply acting out or bad behaviour. We now know that ADHD has biological origins and is a serious medical condition. This book and others like it are crucial in changing the narrative surrounding ADHD because, regrettably, beliefs that ADHD is a result of "bad parenting" still exist today.

An estimated 9.8%, or 6 million U.S. children ages 3–17 have received a diagnosis of ADHD based on data from 2016–2019 (CDC, 2022). The rates of diagnosis peak between the ages of 6 and 11, with around 10% diagnosed, and between ages 12 and 17, with around 13% diagnosed.

ADHD rates also differ significantly by gender and race. Boys are nearly twice as likely as girls to receive an ADHD diagnosis. Black and white children have considerably higher diagnosis rates compared to Hispanic and Asian

American youth (CDC, 2022). The prevalence also varies quite a bit depending on the U.S. state, with estimates ranging from 6% to as high as 16% for current diagnoses. Treatment rates for those diagnosed differ as well, from a low of 58% receiving ADHD treatment in some states to a high of 92% in others.

ADHD Types

Not all ADHD is the same. There are actually three main "presentations" or types of ADHD (CDC, 2023; John Hopkins Medicine, n.d.):

Primarily inattentive: If your teen has this type, their main challenge is focus, organization, and short-term memory. They probably struggle with things like completing tasks, paying attention during conversations or lectures at school, keeping their desk and room tidy, or remembering what assignments are due when.

Primarily hyperactive/impulsive: For this ADHD type, your teen battles more with sitting still, staying quiet when needed, and impulsive behaviour like interrupting others or making spur-of-the-moment (sometimes risky) choices. Their brain gets bored easily, and they may feel restless all the time.

Combined presentation: Some people show strong symptoms in both the inattention/disorganization and hyperactivity/impulsivity realms at similar levels. If your teen has this type, they will struggle with focusing and sitting still. It's tough to get work done, and they may feel constantly distracted while also acting very impulsively and restlessly.

The type of ADHD your teen has can actually change over time, too. When they are younger, you may see more hyperactive traits. These might mellow out as they reach their later teens. Or the opposite can happen where they become more inattentive with age. There's no "right" way for your teen's ADHD to look.

Activity 1: Quiz to Identify Your Teen's Type

Now that you know what the different kinds of ADHD are, you can help your teen figure out which type of ADHD they have. Encourage them to take the following quiz with you.

Instructions: Read each statement in both lists carefully and answer honestly.

Primarily inattentive: Does your teen

- Have trouble staying focused during class lectures or long conversations?
- Feel restless and fidgety a lot?
- Make impulsive decisions without thinking through the consequences?
- Have trouble sitting still during meals or study time?
- Have a tough time remembering deadlines or appointments?

Primarily hyperactive/impulsive: Does your teen

- often misplace things like their keys, wallet, or assignments?
- Have a hard time waiting their turn to talk or interrupt others frequently?
- Usually, have a very disorganized desk and bedroom.
- Blurt out answers before questions have been fully

asked?

- Feel the need to constantly move when they should be still?

If you answered yes to all or most of the first list, then they are likely to have primarily inattentive ADHD. If you answered yes to all or most of the second list, then they are likely to have primarily hyperactive/impulsive ADHD. If they answered yes to a mixture of both lists, then they likely have combined ADHD.

Take some time to think about the different things that your teen struggles with, and make some notes in the space below. You can return to this list again and again as you work through the rest of the book.

Common Traits and Challenges

While ADHD can look different depending on your child's specific type and symptoms, most teens with ADHD struggle with some combination of the following core issues:

- **Impulsivity:** For those with ADHD, it's really tough to think before you act. Your teen may blurt things out without considering if they might be rude or inappropriate. Or they take new risks without weighing the potential downsides. It can hurt friendships and even physical safety to not be able to control those knee-jerk impulses.
- **Distractibility:** If every little thing catches your attention, it's nearly impossible to stay focused,

right? ADHD minds crave stimulation, which makes it easy to zero in on anything new rather than the task or conversation at hand. Squirrels, classmates gossiping, the clock ticking—it all pulls their concentration away.

- **Disorganization:** Keeping track of assignments, notes, their schedule, and household stuff like laundry can feel impossible. ADHD affects the executive functioning skills that handle planning, time management, and overall organization. Days blend together, and your teen will constantly lose track of essential items.
- **Hyperactivity:** Excess energy comes as a standard for the ADHD operating system. Your teen is always itching to move or talk. Sitting relatively still to eat, study, or focus at school goes totally against their nature. While not all ADHD includes hyperactivity, it is super common.

So, which of those core challenges does your teen relate to most? Take notes below on the ADHD traits that feel especially tough day to day.

Activity 2: Which Traits Affect Your Teen Most

Now that you've learned about some of the key traits and challenges those with ADHD face take a minute with your teen to reflect on which resonates most with them.

Instructions: Re-read the explanations of impulsivity, distractibility, disorganization, and hyperactivity above. Then, rank the traits below in order from #1 (most challenging) to #4 (least challenging).

#__Impulsivity

#__Distractibility

#__Disorganization

#__Hyperactivity

After your rankings, use the space below to write 3–5 sentences on how that #1 trait impacts your teen's daily life. Think of specific examples, like losing track of time doing homework because they kept getting distracted. Encourage them to be honest about their struggles!

Knowing your teen's toughest ADHD symptoms can help you both set goals for areas you want to work on with them. We'll keep coming back to these core challenges in future chapters.

The Role of Family in Diagnosis

Getting an ADHD diagnosis for your child can be difficult, but as a parent, you play a critical role in this. By closely observing your child's behaviour at home, tracking their development, and communicating concerns to their doctors and the school, you pave the pathway to getting your kid the support that they desperately need.

It's important to document the challenges your teen faces, like lack of focus, disorganization, forgetfulness, or emotional outbursts. You share these specific examples with your pediatrician to help outline the kinds of care or treatment they need. If your child first exhibits ADHD symptoms at school, then the teachers may be the ones to initially notice an issue. But their impressions, combined with your parental expertise, are what will help medical professionals accurately diagnose ADHD.

You also must advocate for getting your teen proper accommodations and services at school once they are diagnosed. This includes things like preferential seating, extended time on tests, access to counsellors, modified assignments, and behavioural support plans. Not all schools readily provide adequate ADHD assistance, so parents must be proactive and sometimes might have to fight for their child's needs and legal rights.

While getting an ADHD diagnosis can feel overwhelming, remember that you know your child better than anyone else. By giving doctors clear behaviour patterns and pushing the school to offer ADHD resources, you help your teen get the right treatment plan in place. Together with professional support, your love and advocacy will set your kid up for success.

Top Tips for Parents

Here are some top tips for parents newly facing an ADHD diagnosis for their child:

- **Learn all you can about ADHD:** Understanding the signs, symptoms, causes, and treatments will empower you to better support your child.
- **Connect with other parents:** Find local support groups or online communities to exchange advice and encouragement.
- **Communicate with your child:** Explain ADHD in a positive way and emphasize their strengths. Make sure they know you are there for them.
- **Meet with school staff:** Discuss classroom

adaptations and services to meet your child's needs.

- **Try behaviour therapy:** Work on social skills, time management, and organizational habits. Create structure and make sure you use rewards rather than punishment.
- **Establish a medication routine if prescribed:** Note any side effects and adjust the dosage if needed.
- **Foster your child's talents:** Encourage them to develop skills and activities they excel at.
- **Adjust parenting techniques as needed:** Kids with ADHD require lots of patience, flexibility, and creative discipline methods.
- **Adapt household routines to fit your child:** Build in systems and cues to assist with day-to-day tasks.
- **Take care of yourself, too:** Being an advocate, educator, and caregiver is demanding. Make sure to meet your own needs so you can support your child.

ADHD in Key Areas of Teen Life

While ADHD impacts everyone differently, most teens will struggle in some core facets of daily life. Understanding where your child commonly runs into roadblocks can help you provide the targeted support they need.

School Challenges

Academic settings are quite often the most challenging for ADHD brains, with numerous distractions, organization demands, sitting requirements, and boring lectures. You may already be getting lots of notes home about missed assignments, daydreaming in class, or behavioural issues. You can help your teen break big projects down, use planners religiously, leverage focus aids like fidget toys, and frequently communicate with teachers.

Social Struggles

Impulsivity and a lack of focus can make it tough for some ADHD teens to maintain close friendships. They may interrupt others, forget plans, or come across as insensitive. Teach them conversational skills, empathy tactics, how to pick up social cues, and reinforce the value of being a trustworthy friend. Help identify their strengths as well, rather than focusing on all the things they struggle with.

Home Hardships

Juggling chores, routines, family relationships, and homework overwhelms many teens with ADHD who struggle with time blindness, prioritizing, and task initiation. To help them at home, you can set up structured systems for managing tasks and break them into clear step-by-step instructions. Visual lists and charts can be extremely helpful for any age, so think about getting them a diary or a calendar they can pin up to keep track of everything at home. Offer lots of positive reinforcement to combat their negative thinking and celebrate all small wins at home. Patience is essential, too!

It's important to recognize the unique challenges that your child faces in order to help them effectively. However, you should also be aware of their individual strengths in order to offer them the right encouragement and positive reinforcement.

Activity 3: Name Strengths and Challenges

In the space provided below, list your child's unique challenges and strengths in each of these areas:

Key area	Challenges	Strengths
School	• e.g., missed assignments • • • • •	• e.g., great at math • • • • •
Social	• e.g., interrupts others • • • • •	• e.g., loves to help others • • • • •
Home	• e.g., forgets chores • • • • •	• e.g., has lots of hobbies • • • • •

The key is pinpointing your child's ADHD profile—their

unique challenges and strengths. Once you know where they stumble and soar, you can offer the appropriate assistance to set them up for success. The rest of the book will provide you with interactive tips and strategies to help you navigate all three of these areas with your child.

Treatments for ADHD

While ADHD is not something that can be "cured," there are a number of treatment options that you can utilize to help your teen manage their symptoms. Depending on your teen's struggles, you might consider medicating them, or you might choose to focus solely on lifestyle changes and behavioural therapy. Some physicians recommend using both medication and behavioural interventions together for the best results.

Medications

Stimulant medications like Adderall, Concerta, Vyvanse, Ritalin, and others are commonly prescribed to help boost focus, memory, and cognitive control (American Academy of Pediatrics, 2019). Finding the right drug and dosage is tricky, but these meds have been known to help many ADHD patients. It's also important to discuss any side effects openly with the prescribing doctor so you all know what to expect and how to navigate this pathway.

Lifestyle Changes

Certain adjustments can lessen ADHD episodes for some, like getting ample exercise each day, sticking to a routine, limiting distractions, practicing mindfulness techniques, organizing spaces using visual cues, and maintaining a balanced, protein-rich diet (Nigg, 2017). Your teen's executive functioning deficits can be filled in by making structural changes to the home and academic settings.

Behavioural Therapy

Ongoing counselling helps kids practice their vital skills related to impulse control, managing emotions, listening, social dynamics, time management, breaking large assignments into steps, and boosting organization (CDC, 2023). Talk therapy can also help to improve self-esteem issues that are common among ADHD youth.

Coping Strategies

Finally, teach your ADHD teen healthy adaptive techniques for navigating their unique struggles. This can mean walking away when angered, allowing extra travel time for distractedness, asking for written instructions to offset forgetfulness, or using apps to structure studying. Help them learn what calms an ADHD brain. Coping tactics will provide them with lifelong tools.

With patience and a combo plan targeting problematic symptoms, you can help your teen successfully manage their ADHD. Stay observant of their setbacks and progress so you can adjust their support as needed.

Activity 4: Current Treatments

In the space below, note down the things that you are already doing to treat your teen's ADHD and which techniques you might like to try next or alongside what you are currently doing:

Key Takeaways and What's Next

Before we move on to Part 2, let's recap what we covered in this chapter as an overview of ADHD:

- ADHD is a common neurological disorder typically diagnosed in childhood. Core symptoms include inattention, hyperactivity, and impulsivity.
- It impacts about 9.8% of youth, with boys more frequently diagnosed than girls. Diagnosing ADHD requires evaluating behavior patterns.
- The three ADHD subtypes are predominantly inattentive, predominantly hyperactive/impulsive, and combined. Identifying your teen's subtype helps guide their treatment.
- Common challenges those with ADHD face involve distractibility, disorganization, interrupting, restlessness, emotional dysregulation, and following multi-step directions.
- Treatments include stimulant medications to improve focus, behavioural therapy to teach coping mechanisms, and lifestyle changes like more exercise.
- As a parent, you play a huge role in getting your child accurately diagnosed, advocating for school accommodations, reinforcing positive behaviours, and helping implement management strategies at home.

Coming up, we'll go deeper into common ADHD struggles around executive functioning, social skills, managing emotions, and building self-confidence. You'll discover targeted activities and interventions to help your teen minimize their daily struggles. I want to provide the knowledge and tools that you need to help your child feel empowered to embrace their unique ADHD mind.

* * *

PART 2: SCHOOLING WITH ADHD

CHAPTER 2: EXECUTIVE FUNCTIONING AND ADHD

Deficits in executive functions such as planning, categorization, organization, and attention leave them lost amid a sea of things, unable to figure out what to do next. –Randy O. Frost

Jake barely made it to graduation after years of constant friction with his teachers and counsellors. They all criticized his difficulty paying attention in lectures, messy, disorganized assignments, forgetfulness, and missing deadlines time and time again. Over time, Jake internalized this sense of intense self-doubt from feeling constantly berated by his authority figures.

However, Jake's family recognized glimmers of brilliance

in him when he hyperfocused tirelessly on building his complex Minecraft kingdoms for hours. He demonstrated innate talents and creatively leveraged technology to invent and lead communities in the game.

So, despite his underwhelming transcripts, Jake's parents encouraged him to apply to a specialized video game design university, where he could nurture those innate skills. He *thrived*—finally free to immerse himself in the world of programming virtual worlds while also combining storytelling with engineering.

Shortly after graduating, Jake founded a startup company that pioneered immersive mixed-reality simulations. His ADHD traits—boundless imagination, design obsession, and infectious enthusiasm—helped to secure the venture capital, and very soon, the industry's top talent rapidly began to realize his entrepreneurial vision.

Today, as Jake's company prepares for a hugely successful IPO, he speaks openly about channelling his ADHD strengths to meet the modern workforce's increasing demand for innovation. Jake's resilience in pursuing his professional calling, *despite* his discouraging academic experiences and his early executive functioning struggles, highlights the possibilities that are available when a teen's neurodivergence and strengths are embraced.

What Is Executive Functioning?

Executive function is like the boss of your teen's brain—it's in charge of overseeing everything and making sure tasks get handled properly. It's that voice of reason that tells them to wait their turn instead of shouting out the answer in class. It reminds them that they need to leave for school earlier since they always forget a book in their locker. It helps them break a big homework assignment down into smaller action steps.

Essentially, executive functioning is a set of mental management skills that let all of us organize information, pay attention, switch focus, plan ahead, use time wisely, remember details, avoid saying whatever pops into our heads, and learn from past choices that didn't go so well (Belsky, 2019).

Some of the main components of executive functioning include (Belsky, 2019; Belsky, n.d.; Diamond, 2013):

- **Working memory:** This is what enables your teen to store information for quick recall, which is vital for things like taking notes in biology class, grasping math formulas during a lecture, or remembering the rules of a game their friends are playing.
- **Inhibitory control:** This mental skill allows your teen to stop themselves from acting impulsively, like not shouting out the Jeopardy answer early or thinking before they fire off a snarky text to your friend.
- **Cognitive flexibility:** This lets your teen adjust their behaviour or thinking to changing situations. For example, transitioning from lounging over summer break to sitting attentively in classes again.
- **Task initiation:** Here, your teen's brain plans the steps needed to get going on assignments or responsibilities and pushes them into action vs. procrastinating.
- **Organization:** This is how your teen organizes

info into understandable categories and prioritizes what's most important to focus on—like sorting class notes or keeping their locker neat.

How ADHD Impacts Executive Function

When your teen has ADHD, those executive functioning skills that help them juggle all the expectations of school, home, friends, and growing up don't work quite right. They likely struggle with the following (ADDA Editorial Team, 2023; Koseva, 2022):

- **Prioritizing:** Is studying for that math test more urgent than organizing their locker? Calculating importance is tough when everything feels like a crisis!
- **Time perception:** Estimating how long assignments will take or how much time has passed is tricky and can cause your teen chronic lateness. Due dates seem to sneak up on them.
- **Getting started:** Getting started means overcoming inertia, which can feel impossible some days. Your teen will delay, freeze, or distract themselves while waiting for the motivation fairy—who doesn't actually exist.
- **Breaking down instructions:** Multi-step directions will completely overwhelm them. Planning the steps between writing up a paper or starting a project can feel really daunting.
- **Organization:** Orderliness helps us all access information quickly, but papers pile up, and your teen's room is chaos central, no matter how often

you nag them.

- **Controlling reactions:** Impulse control is hard when every thought that pops into their head instantly comes out of their mouths, even if it's silly or rude.
- **Planning ahead:** Hmm, what's due tomorrow or next Friday? Predicting future responsibilities, budgeting money, or mapping goals over months doesn't come naturally to ADHD teens.
- **Remembering obligations:** You asked them to take out the garbage, their friend wants her book back, and they had plans to play the Xbox tonight with friends—all of these tasks were forgotten in favour of scrolling through TikTok.

Executive functioning impairment makes managing life's daily expectations super frustrating—both for you and your teen. Now that you know the issues, we'll dig into workarounds.

The Link Between Executive Function and ADHD

Brain imaging research shows that executive functioning skills like self-control, working memory, and mental flexibility all happen in the frontal lobes of the brain (Diamond, 2013). Guess which part shows less activity in those with ADHD? Yep—that same region!

Specifically, decreased dopamine and norepinephrine in that frontal area throw off connections between brain networks managing concentration, planning, and regulating emotions (Hunt, n.d.). The resulting executive function deficiencies then exacerbate common ADHD behaviour symptoms.

It becomes a vicious cycle where ADHD creates executive function weaknesses around things like attention, organization, and impulse control. Those executive function problems then lead to more severe ADHD symptoms. The worse your ADHD gets, the weaker your executive functioning skills become.

For example, low dopamine makes it hard to initiate starting homework. So, your teen keeps putting it off until the last minute. Then, their rushed, chaotic homework efforts are so much less efficient, and they get distracted easily without finishing. Frustrated, they impulsively toss their books off the bed. Do you see the ongoing loop your kid is getting stuck in?

But don't lose hope! While it's true that you can't rewrite the neural wiring your teen was born with, you *can* help them learn coping skills to improve their focus, planning, and self-regulation. Strengthening their executive functioning makes managing their ADHD symptoms much more possible!

Importance of Strengthening Executive Functioning Skills

So, you now understand that ADHD poses executive functioning challenges for your teen. But don't resign yourself to the fact that this is their fate forever. With some effort on both your parts, you *can* improve their self-management abilities and help to make school and life flow better for them.

When your teen boosts their executive function capabilities, they'll reap rewards like:

- **Better academic outcomes:** Staying organized, blocking out distractions, managing time, and completing long-term projects effectively means they will achieve better grades!
- **Improved life skills:** Outside school, they'll handle personal obligations more responsibly, whether it's sticking to club commitments or just getting themselves to bed on time.
- **More reliable and responsible:** Since they'll better regulate their impulses, wait their turn patiently, and think before reacting, people will see them as more trustworthy and mature.
- **Greater independence:** When they can juggle schedules, break big jobs into steps, and push past barriers to get started, they'll need less oversight from parents and teachers guiding them through their responsibilities.

Who doesn't want more self-control, personal success, a positive reputation, and freedom? Investing in strengthening your teen's mental management skills now pays off with a solid foundation for their future.

Let's look at where your teen's executive deficits are the greatest so we can decide what to address first now that we understand what executive function is, how ADHD affects it, and the advantages of improving these skills.

Activity 5: Identify Your Executive Function Strengths and Weaknesses

Let's figure out which executive functioning components are toughest for your teen. This quiz highlights the common areas that ADHD can impair. Remind your teen to be honest in checking off the challenges they face so we can then work to improve those skills.

- I have trouble getting started on homework, chores, or tasks, even though I want to get them done.
- I regularly misplace things like coats, shoes, and class supplies even though they have a "designated spot."
- I don't realize how much time passes when gaming, reading, or chatting with friends.
- I often forget what tasks my parents or teachers have asked me to do.
- I tend to interrupt people mid-conversation because I can't wait my turn.
- I usually underestimate how long assignments will take and end up rushing at the last minute.
- My bookbag, desktop, and locker are incredibly disorganized, no matter how often I tidy up.
- I make impulsive choices in the moment that I later wish I could take back.

After checking the areas your teen struggles with, circle the top three executive functioning challenges you want to tackle first.

Activity 6: Setting Executive Function Goals

Now that you've identified your teen's top executive functioning challenges, let's talk about a game plan!

Take the three challenges you circled from the checklist. Write each one in the spaces below. Then, brainstorm two or three specific, measurable goals for improving each of those three key areas this school quarter.

Take a look at the following example to help you:

Challenge:	I struggle to get started on tasks
Goals:	• begin two tasks before noon every weekday • set 30 min timer and work nonstop • ask parents to check in on progress

Now, fill in the following chart tailored to your three challenges:

Challenge #1:	
Goals to improve:	• • •
Challenge #2:	
Goals to improve:	• • •
Challenge #3:	
Goals to improve:	• • •

Be sure to help your teen make their goals super specific, like "practice starting essays 2x a week" rather than vague plans like "procrastinate less." Also, focus on small, tangible wins rather than big, intimidating milestones. Check back on their progress every two weeks and celebrate even the smallest milestones with them. Remember, positive reinforcement is so important!

Key Takeaways and What's Next

Let's recap what we learned about executive functioning and ADHD:

- Executive functioning refers to critical management skills like organization, focus, planning, and impulse control. They help your teen effectively meet life's demands.
- Core executive functions include working memory, inhibition control, cognitive flexibility, and task initiation.
- Due to shared neural pathway deficiencies, ADHD and executive dysfunction go hand in hand.
- Common problems involve getting started, time blindness, breaking down instructions, disorganization, emotional outbursts, and forgetfulness.
- Boosting executive skills leads to academic and life success.
- We identified your teen's personal executive function challenges and set goals to help them improve.

In the next chapter, we'll build on your teen's strengths to develop customized systems for conquering those executive function challenges. You'll discover learning techniques that are tailored to how your teen's unique ADHD mind works best. Get ready to help them really thrive!

CHAPTER 3: DISCOVER YOUR STRENGTHS AND UNDERSTAND YOUR WEAKNESSES

Accept yourself, your strengths, your weaknesses, your truths, and know what tools you have to fulfill your purpose. –Steve Maraboli

ADHD Superpowers

While ADHD certainly comes with its challenges, the unique wiring of your teen's brain also brings certain superpowers! People with ADHD often excel in areas like (ADDitude Editors, 2016b; Burch, 2022):

- **Creativity:** Your teen might be able to make unexpected connections between ideas, approaching problems from totally different angles than their peers. That ingenuity translates well into the arts, writing, and visionary thinking.
- **Curiosity:** Your teen's inquisitive nature often leads them to ask *lots* of questions. This might get frustrating sometimes, but it can unlock new discoveries and interesting conversations. They retain information best when their learning is active like this.
- **Humour:** Your teen tends to appreciate and wield humour and wit effortlessly to boost morale and form connections. Laughter comes easily to them.
- **Energetic:** Your teen's vibrant zest for life is infectious. They dive fully into activities and can motivate others with enthusiastic passion.
- **Empathy:** Collaborate with classmates whom you connect with emotionally. Study groups with friends feel rewarding, thanks to your emotional intuition. Help uplift peers who struggle, too.

By leveraging these innate superpowers, people with ADHD can find great success following passions in areas like entrepreneurship, athletics, music, writing, science, comedy, and more!

Did You Know?

Celebrities like musician Justin Timberlake, gymnast Simone Biles, comedian Howie Mandel, inventor Thomas Edison, and author Terry Pratchett have all thrived hugely while managing ADHD (ADDitude Editors, 2016a; *Famous People With ADHD,* 2022). Like them, your teen can channel their strengths into awesome achievements, too!

Leveraging ADHD Superpowers

So, how can you help your teen use these superpowers to help them in school and with their executive functions?

- **Creativity:** They can use their ingenuity to make learning engaging by drawing colourful diagrams, maps, and sketches to illustrate different concepts. They might also create silly rhymes or acronyms to memorize definitions.
- **Curiosity:** Your teen can harness their inquisitiveness by exploring subject matters deeply through additional reading or videos beyond the minimum school requirements. Let their interests guide them to deeper learning.
- **Humour:** They might turn boring lectures or dense textbook chapters into crafty cartoons or witty commentary related to the content. The comic relief will boost their information retention!
- **Energetic:** They can burn restless energy by actively highlighting texts, crafting flashcards to quiz themselves, or converting notes into songs while studying. Excess energy can fuel focus when it's channelled productively.

- **Empathy:** Collaborate with classmates whom you connect with emotionally. Study groups with friends feel rewarding, thanks to your emotional intuition. Help uplift peers who struggle, too.

Playing to these strengths not only makes schoolwork more engaging but also builds executive function skills in the process—like sustaining focus, converting instructions into tactical steps, practicing organization through note-taking and illustrations, and expanding working memory capabilities.

Help your teen put their ADHD brainpower to work for them in managing both assignments *and* symptoms! You never know; they might just be the next Justin Timberlake.

Activity 7: Map Superpowers

Let's uncover the special ADHD skills and talents that make your teen who they are! Here, spend some time reflecting on moments where they shined or received praise from teachers, parents, coaches, and so on.

Instructions: In the space below, write 2-3 strengths or talents that come naturally to your teen. They can be things like creativity, empathy, determination, writing ability, musicality, athleticism, leadership, enthusiasm, or anything else they excel at.

Then, for each one, think about how they currently apply them at school, at home, or in extracurriculars. Finally, consider how they can apply these skills going forward —think of their future career, relationships, or other life domains; this is the "big picture" of how these skills can help your teen thrive.

They might need some help looking at the big picture; give them some examples, but encourage them to think for themselves here rather than giving them the answer. They might be pleasantly surprised at how skilled they really are!

Strength #1:

How it is currently applied:

How to apply it in the future:

Strength #2:

How it is currently applied:

How to apply it in the future:

Strength #3:

How it is currently applied:

How to apply it in the future:

ADHD Kryptonite

Along with your teen's absolute brilliance also come common ADHD pitfalls that might trip them up sometimes, too. They may struggle in zones like (Hurley, 2016; Mayo Clinic Staff, 2023):

- **Distractibility:** Squirrels outside, pen clicking, classmates whispering... little disruptions pull their attention constantly, making concentrating on lessons or homework next to impossible! They miss important instructions and content while their focus ping-pongs around other things.
- **Forgetfulness:** Birthdays, assignments, where their shoes are—dates and details just fall straight out of their overwhelmed working memory. People might sometimes think they're thoughtless, but the truth is they genuinely miss or lose track of crucial information and are always playing catch-up.
- **Hyperfocusing:** When activities truly captivate you, like gaming or chatting with friends, you tunnel your vision and become oblivious to anything else going on for hours. Time flies by, and other obligations are forgotten until the hyperfocus lifts, leaving unfinished priorities behind.

A teen I worked with—we'll call him James—once told me how his hyperfocus tendency made him lose track of time and assignments:

"I will become so engrossed in watching failed videos on YouTube that I will forget to begin this enormous English paper that is due tomorrow." The next thing I knew, it was 10 p.m., and I hadn't eaten dinner or done any homework. Then, I am in a complete state of haste, working through the night to complete the task as soon as possible. It's like I'm powerless to break myself out of the hyperfocus trance... no matter the chaos waiting on the other side."

ADHD pitfalls can be tough! What can you do to help your teen navigate them?

Leverage Your Strengths to Overcome Weaknesses

The key to succeeding with ADHD lies in optimizing natural abilities to overcome any weaknesses. With the right encouragement and confidence, your teen can use their strengths to overcome their weaknesses.

For example, they can harness that restless energy through:

- Physical exercise: Instead of fidgeting in class, encourage your teen to join the soccer or track team. They'll expend those buckets of energy while practicing drills, sprints, and skills. Sports are great for engrossing hyperactive minds.
- Creative pursuits: They could pour all that mental restlessness into theatre improv, learning guitar, painting anime characters, or journaling poetry. The arts have been known to satisfy the craving for stimulation.
- Passion projects: Alternatively, they might dive fully into self-directed interests like video editing, website design, botany experiments, or whatever fun thing engages their curiosity! Allow them to hyperfocus on what captivates them.

There are many ways in which your teen can make the most of their strengths to overcome their weaknesses.

Let's look at a few more examples before you start thinking about their individual weaknesses. They could:

- Use their humour and personability to make study groups entertaining instead of dull snoozefests.
- Use their creativity to make to-do lists more fun and motivating by using colourful pens, stickers, illustrations, and so on.
- Harness their energetic nature by taking frequent active standing or movement breaks while doing homework—stretching, bouncing on an exercise ball, or dancing to music periodically.
- Let their innate curiosity guide their schoolwork, like papers and projects—encourage them to follow tangents that fascinate them, even if it's not required.
- Use their empathy superpower during group assignments by encouraging their struggling teammates, asking them how they prefer to contribute, and recognizing their skills.
- Counteract their distractibility by choosing workspaces selectively—like their quiet bedroom over the noisy kitchen.
- Resist hyperfocus from derailing their responsibilities by setting alarms to take breaks, then setting new alarms reminding them to return to their tasks.

Remember, ADHD isn't a flaw; it's just an alternate way of thinking day-to-day. Your teen can use the strengths that they outlined earlier in the chapter to overcome their weaknesses creatively by developing systems that function with how their unique mind operates. The key is helping them match their functional coping mechanisms to their personal profile—exactly what we're going to do next!

Activity 8: Map Pitfalls

Let's evaluate when and where ADHD kryptonite typically strikes your teen. By pinpointing their biggest impediments, you can help them strategize potential solutions.

Instructions: In Column 1 below, write 2–3 examples of your teen's forgetfulness, distraction, hyperfocusing, or other executive functioning weaknesses. In Column 2, describe the situation where that weakness tends to arise. Finally, in Column 3, brainstorm an initial idea for overcoming that hurdle using strength as leverage. You can use the examples in the last section to help you come up with some ideas here.

Weakness	**When it emerges**	**Plan to overcome**
e.g., forget due dates	Big school projects with lots of moving pieces spread out over the weeks	Use creative checklists and reminders

Key Takeaways and What's Next

Let's recap what we have covered so far about capitalizing on your teen's strengths while managing their weaknesses:

- ADHD minds have strengths like creativity, curiosity, humour, passion, empathy, and energy.
- You can connect their natural abilities to success in school, hobbies, relationships, and careers.
- However, pitfalls like distraction, forgetfulness, and hyperfocus still hinder them at times.
- Identify when or where they struggle specifically and make plans to counteract using their strengths.
- For example, harness energy through exercise versus fidgeting. Or set phone timers to break hyperfocus.
- Play to their innate skills and aptitude to neutralize and navigate weaknesses.

Now that you know your teen's personal ADHD superpowers and kryptonite trouble spots, we'll start to dig into concrete organizational systems, schedules, and planning tactics. It's time to channel that untamed mental energy toward school achievement and executive function mastery.

* * *

CHAPTER 4: GET ORGANIZED

> *Organizing isn't about perfection; it's about efficiency, reducing stress and clutter, saving time and money, and improving your overall quality of life. –Christina Scalise*

Why Organization Matters

As you probably know by now, organization doesn't come naturally to neurodivergent minds (Koseva, 2023). However, establishing and maintaining structure can truly elevate how well your teen functions. Implementing systems for their stuff, schedules, and spaces creates order amidst their ADHD chaos.

The benefits of being organized include

- finding important items like devices, glasses, and assignment notes fast instead of frenzied hunting.
- Reduced chronic lateness since gears, coats, and bags have designated homes.

- Less overwhelmed and frustrated scrambling to meet deadlines or obligations.
- More confidence in handling responsibilities independently.
- More mental energy since they are not constantly playing catch-up.
- Focus is freed up for learning versus repeatedly reorganizing.

Whereas living amidst ongoing disarray sabotages your teen's success through

- lost homework buried under a pile of clutter.
- Forgetting commitments without calendars.
- No clean clothes from overflowing hampers.
- Misplaced keys, making them late yet again!

Simply put, when your teen is surrounded by too much turmoil, their brain is kind of short-circuit. Helping them establish structure helps them operate optimally.

Organizing Physical Space

First, let's tackle organizing the key spaces your teen occupies and making them anxiety-free! Start by looking at their bedroom, backpack, and locker to help them streamline their efficiency.

Activity 9: Assess Personal Spaces

Okay, let's evaluate how organized your teen's everyday environments currently are using a simple 1–5 scale:

Bedroom

1. Utter chaos
2. Pretty messy
3. Some order
4. Mostly neat
5. Extremely organized

Current rating: __

Backpack

1. Total pit of doom
2. Lots of loose papers
3. Some main folders
4. Mostly structured
5. Thoughtfully streamlined

Current rating: __

Locker

1. Yikes biohazard!
2. Random everything
3. Some order in chaos
4. Tidier lately
5. Everything has a perfect place

Current rating: __

Now that you have your teen's ratings, you can streamline which areas need to be prioritized first. Take a look at the following tips for each area:

Bedroom tips:

- Use shelf bins, stacks of shoe boxes, and underbed containers to categorize clothes, tech accessories, sports equipment, and so on—labelling helps!
- Designate wall hooks for coats, hats, and bags close to the door for grab-and-go ease.
- Shelve books, video games, and DVDs rather than having them in floor piles.
- Assign a small crate, tray, or basket for items that move around, like chargers, watches, and wallets.

Backpack tips:

- Have colour-coded 2-pocket folders for each academic subject. Encourage them to regularly file their papers and handouts.
- Get them a pencil case stocked with writing, marking, and erasing tools, plus a calculator, mini stapler, and any other equipment so their items don't get jumbled among everything else.
- Encourage them to clean out and reorganize their backpack weekly or biweekly.

Locker tips:

- Use small shelf organizers for textbooks, devices, and other supplies.
- They can use magnetic clips to attach schedules, reminders, photos, and others to the interior walls.
- Using a mini whiteboard lets them write notes for themselves.

- Locker shelf bins provide vertical storage.
- Encourage them to declutter regularly.

Jot down two or three initial ideas below for how you and your teen plan to improve their structure and efficiency based on the tips above:

When you break decluttering and organizing stuff down into small, doable steps, your teen will find the whole concept much less stressful and overwhelming. They will quickly reap the benefits of an organized space, and that will motivate them to maintain it. Just focus on making small, sustainable changes over time.

Organizing Time

ADHD and time blindness tend to go hand-in-hand. Whether your teen is losing track of hours passed or underestimating how long their tasks require, the fact is that they lack an internal clock. So, helping them to create external time organizers is essential!

Activity 10: Evaluate Time Management

Let's start by assessing where your teen currently is with their time management. On a scale of 1–5, rate how consistently your teen implements each time organization tool:

Planner/agenda:

1. Never use one
2. Sometimes, write assignments down

3. Record major due dates fairly regularly
4. Detail most obligations and appointments
5. Comprehensively maps days

Current rating: __

Checklists:

1. What are those?
2. Occasionally make a to-do list
3. Check off some tasks during busier days
4. Create daily lists but not always fully completed
5. Break their day into line items and check them all off

Current rating: __

Alarms:

1. Their phone alarms are always snoozed or dismissed
2. They set a few alerts but often ignore them
3. They have some alarms for key times
4. Use alarms fairly regularly
5. Strategically use alarms to structure their day

Current rating: __

Now that you know which areas your teen could use some help in, take a look at the tips below and think about how you can incorporate some of these into their lives to help streamline their time management.

Planners/agendas:

Encouraging your teen to map all their obligations, assignments, practices, meets, appointments, and so on visually makes juggling everything much less overwhelming for them. Take them shopping and buy a paper planner, diary, or calendar, or they can use a digital calendar to:

- Record homework, project, and test due dates as soon as they are assigned.
- Block off regular obligations like yearbooks, youth groups, or part-time jobs.
- Enter special events and social plans as they arise.
- Build accountability by seeing everything consolidated.

Wall calendars:

Hang a large calendar centrally at home to maintain an overview of their bigger trimester or semester schedule. Mark tests, travel, school breaks, and even family plans.

Checklists:

Break each day down into specific to-do lists so your teen can methodically accomplish their tasks. Checking stuff off will help motivate them and give them a dopamine hit (Davis, n.d.).

Alarms:

Use your phone, watches, timers, and apps to ping reminders to start tasks, take breaks, end screen time, commence bedtime routines, and anything else. Alerts can act as an anchor against timeblindness.

Discuss some time-management goals with your teen tailored to their weak spots and jot them down in the space provided below:

By recording information externally, your teen can compensate for their internal executive functioning gaps.

Organizing Schedules

With all your teens' stuff and time management organized, let's now optimize their actual schedule! Carefully plotting out their recurring obligations can help them immensely in their school career. The goal is to help stop them from feeling constantly frenzied and behind all the time and to take more initiative in taking back control of their schedules.

Activity 11: Assess Schedule Skills

You know the drill by now! On a scale of 1–5, rate how consistently your teen implements the following schedule organization elements:

Obligation mapping:

1. Their calendar is empty
2. Major stuff makes it onto the calendar sometimes
3. They schedule some events and assignments
4. They are pretty good at tracking their activities
5. Meticulously document all obligations

Current rating: __

Designated study times:

1. What's that?
2. Occasionally, plan study sessions
3. Try to study on the same days but at no set times
4. Schedule weekly study blocks usually honoured
5. Strategically block-set homework and study times

Current rating: __

Buffer transitions:

1. Always running late!
2. Build in small buffers but still often late
3. Realistic buffers for some obligations
4. Carefully schedule transition time
5. Master at buffers, so never rush!

Current rating: __

Which area is your teen struggling in the most here? Take a look at the following tips for each area.

Mapping commitments:

Encourage them to transfer what's mapped in their planner or posted on wall calendars into a master weekly schedule template. This overview lets them visualize blocks of demanding classes, heavy extracurriculars, or work shifts. This way, they can see the whole picture in one place.

Block study time:

Your teen could pencil in regular one- to two-hour homework chunks on lighter days without many fixed activities. Treat study sessions exactly like a sports practice that they will never miss! Keeping it consistent overrides their procrastination temptation—you can even think about offering a reward or something to look forward to afterward.

Buffer transitions:

ADHD brains struggle to estimate how long moving between schoolwork, errands, and sports practice actually takes while accounting for traffic, pitstops, and other things. Teach them to schedule 30- to 60-minute buffers so they don't arrive late all the time.

Based on the tips above, make some notes on specific ideas you are planning to incorporate with your teen in the space below:

Make time to sit and review your teen's schedule with them weekly at first, encouraging them to make edits as needed. Ultimately, they will begin to internalize the predictable rhythms of their schedule and will minimize the day-to-day decision-making and surprises that used to overwhelm them!

Overcoming Barriers to Organization

Sure, the organization sounds good in theory. But between ADHD paralysis and unsupportive environments, it often crumbles in reality. Let's close out this chapter by taking a look at some helpful tips for getting unstuck when overwhelmed takes hold.

Getting Unstuck

When your teen is facing a disastrous bedroom or an avalanche of homework papers, they're often tempted to shut down, close the door, and find something else to do. But you can help them take small steps:

- Set a short timer and encourage them to work intensely for just 10–15 minutes and accomplish whatever is possible within that time frame. They'll be surprised how much they can get done in that short amount of time, and it will boost their momentum instead of reinforcing the urge to give up entirely.
- Go in and help them! You can chat while tackling the decluttering together. You can make it social and fun.
- Listen to their favourite pumped-up playlist while organizing. Upbeat music can help anyone overcome inertia and resistance.

Structure Around Others

Between messy family members or households with limited storage options, maintaining organization can feel impossible if other people or spaces constantly work against your teen. Try

- Using creative storage hacks like over-the-door hanging shelves or under-bed organizers to carve out tidy spaces.
- Using checklists so essential items have designated areas.

- Encouraging everyone to take responsibility for their own spaces within a messy home.

Look for compromises and control what you can to create orderly environments that promote focus despite any surrounding chaos!

Key Takeaways and What's Next

Let's recap what we covered about getting organized:

- Organizations benefit ADHD brains by reducing overwhelming feelings and clutter distraction.
- Tackle physical spaces first, like streamlining their bedroom, backpack, and locker.
- Use planning tools to structure your time around obligations and study blocks.
- Create consistent homes for your teen's stuff and systems guiding things back to proper places.
- Schedule obligations and transition buffers realistically.
- Break inertia by timer-targeting tasks and inviting accountability.

Next, let's build customized study strategies that maximize focus and retention based on how your teen's unique mind best absorbs and engages with material. We're going to play to those neurodivergent strengths to help school feel more exciting and less exhausting!

* * *

CHAPTER 5: KNOW YOUR STUDY STYLE

When we build on our strengths and daily successes — instead of focusing on failures — we simply learn more. – Tom Rath

Activity 12: Learning Style Quiz

Not all students absorb information the same way. Determining whether your teen learns better visually, auditorily, by reading and writing, or through hands-on action helps them customize their study plans for ultimate information retention.

In this activity, we will uncover your teen's personal learning preferences! For each statement below, ask them to rank how true that approach sounds from 1 (not me at all) to 5 (yes, exactly me!).

Statement	**1**	**2**	**3**	**4**	**5**
Visual					

I remember better using images, charts, or concept maps					
Following video tutorials makes sense to me.					
I prefer teachers who use a whiteboard, slides or props.					
Auditory **Listening to lectures sticks better than reading alone.**					
Recording myself repeating facts helps retention.					
Making up songs or acronyms works well for memorizing things.					
Reading/writing **I take very detailed notes from textbook readings.**					
Re-writing facts in my own words cements my understanding.					
Hands-on action **Doing experiments, model building, or simulations works well.**					

I study the best pacing while reciting concepts out loud.					
I retain most when I am able to be active in applying knowledge.					

Now, take a look at which area your teen scored highest, and you should be able to figure out which style of learning suits them the best.

We're going to explore each learning style in depth now, with tips and tricks to help your teen make the most of their unique learning style.

Visual Learners

If visuals resonate most with your teen when absorbing new information, then embrace that! You can help them optimize graphic-heavy studying through the following techniques (Columbia State Community College, n.d.-b.; Fleming, 2018a):

Diagrams, charts, and concept maps: They shouldn't just copy words from the chalkboard; encourage them to reinterpret lectures and textbook sections. They can put their notes into colourful sketches that map out key ideas, their relationships, and their sequences. Images will stick better when this is your teen's learning style!

Colour coding: They could use highlighters, pens, and markers to differentiate concepts, highlight essential definitions, and embed visual interest across their notes and handouts. The vibrant visual expression will help to keep them engaged in their learning.

Process drawings: Illustrate sequences like the water cycle, how bills become laws, geometric proofs, and so on, in multi-step panels like a comic strip. Artistically walking through workflows helps cement their understanding.

Video demos: YouTube offers unlimited tutorials demonstrating everything from calculus strategies to making crepes! Search "[topic] + how-to" with them whenever written explanations baffle them—they can watch experts in action instead!

Keep studying lively for your teen's visual ADHD brain! They can creatively convert their learning content into memorable graphics, colour-splashed outlines, and dynamic videos—textbooks can't compete with that excitement!

Auditory Learners

If your teen retains the information well through listening and speaking, then you can help them put those auditory strengths to work! They can maximize their sound-centered studying via (Columbia State Community College, n.d.-b; Fleming, 2018b):

Verbal review: Your teen can digest dense textbook sections by first reading silently and then verbally summarizing the main ideas out loud. Speaking the content helps them to solidify the meanings versus just trying to do so inside their heads.

Lecture replay: They could record their teacher's lectures and sample problems and then replay audio while they're out walking the dog, folding laundry, or doing other mundane tasks. They can even replay the lesson as many times as they want.

Talk it out: Physically speaking, concepts, steps, and definitions actually activate different neural pathways, which helps to build your teen's retention. Get them to talk through complicated math problems instead of trying to do it in their heads.

Songs and rhymes: From grammar rules in rhyming lyrics to mathematical sequences in song melodies, silly mnemonic devices can help to make memorizing dry information much more fun. Upbeat auditory gimmicks are known to boost focus, too.

If your teen's ADHD brain is wired to tune into podcasts and music easily, encourage them to harness that power in other auditory ways.

Reading/Writing Learners

For those teens who naturally retain information through reading and writing, you can help them to play to their strengths by encouraging the following techniques (Bay Atlantic University, 2022; *Guide for reading & writing learners,* n.d.):

Annotation: Instead of passively reading, your teen can actively engage with their textbooks by highlighting major points, underlining definitions, starring key terms, and scribbling notes in the margins.

Handwritten notes: They can fully immerse themselves in their learning by using physical paper notebooks for note-taking during lectures. The cognitive effort of manually writing out ideas helps solidify their memory.

Flashcards: Writing vocabulary words, historical names, formula elements, or anything else that needs to be memorized on portable flashcards lets your teen review them anytime, whether they're killing time in lines or rides between sports practices.

Summaries: Instead of just glossing through chapters, encourage your teen to pause periodically while reading to verbally summarize the main points or write them down in a single paragraph. Articulating and paraphrasing information builds their overall comprehension.

Your teen's natural reading and writing neurological sequence can guide them in absorbing textbook and teacher content, helping them to fortify their understanding.

Kinesthetic Learners

Hands-on ADHD learners absorb concepts best through moving, building, and interactive exercises. Help your teen incorporate that tactile learning through the following strategies (Houghton University, 2023; Show Me Images, n.d.):

Tactile aids: They might mould flow charts from clay, stack vocabulary term cubes in categorized towers, or piece together magnetic atom models—hands-on aids bring their study matter alive through touch!

Active breaks: Between notebook pages or textbook chapters, encourage your teen to take a brief break to do some wall pushups or jog in the hallway. This gets their bodies moving, stimulating endorphin surges. A physically re-energized teen is a mentally re-engaged teen.

3D prototypes: Instead of writing down a description of electric circuit components and their interactions, actually build a working model with them! This will leave them with lasting comprehension.

Teach peers: After digesting lessons on historical battles or orchestra instrumentation, they might actively relay that fresh knowledge by teaching it to their friends through role-playing activities.

Let your teen's natural inclination for hands-on learning guide their study methods. Help them to experiment and get creative with it!

Blended Approaches

While everyone tends to have one core learning preference, often using a blended approach to learning can be even more effective for your ADHD teen. By switching between learning styles, you can keep their distracted, impulsive brains engaged for longer and better information retention.

For example, your teen might follow a textbook chapter first by silently reading and highlighting the key passages. Then, they could verbally summarize the most important points into a voice memo while visually sketching a mindmap to connect the ideas.

Later on, your teen might walk through and teach those chapter topics to a friend using their highlighted and annotated book, audio summary, and original drawings as teaching aids. Finally, the pair could then quiz each other with handwritten flashcards they made to identify remaining knowledge gaps.

This kind of blended learning cycle will repetitively expose your teen to information across different learning channels, strengthening the neural connections each way. It also sustains their engagement by regularly shifting activities to maintain their interest in the material—something that might be a real struggle for your ADHD right now.

Activity 13: Overcoming School Struggles

Now that we've learned some new strategies for the different learning styles, let's put it all into practice. Take a look at the common school struggles listed below and spend some time discussing and making notes with your teen about how they can overcome them.

Lecture obstacles: Frequent distraction, forgetting key points, or tuning out long talks.

How can your teen overcome this?

Example answers:

- Doodle concepts to help focus on auditory info.
- Assign peer note-sharing to fill gaps.
- Record the lecture to replay later.
- Build visual maps summarizing key concepts.

Test-taking troubles: Anxiety and executive function gaps cause test performance pitfalls.

How can your teen overcome this?

Example answers:

- Study with online practice quizzes to test their knowledge.
- Recite formulas aloud without notes before exams.
- Review using game show apps to introduce the content repetitively.
- Teach chapters to friends to cement their understanding.

Group project issues: Social dynamics are complicated by your teen's impulsiveness or poor planning, which can aggravate group work.

How can your teen overcome this?

Example answers:

- Use online collaborative spaces to organize research.
- Maintain shared agendas to ensure equal roles.
- Set alarms to keep all partners on the timeline.
- Design visual presentation elements to match everyone's talents.

Key Takeaways and What's Next

Let's recap what we have explored about optimized study strategies:

- Tailor learning approaches to your teen's visual, auditory, reading/writing, or kinesthetic strengths that you were shown through the quiz results.
- Visual learners utilize graphic organizing tools like idea maps, colour-coded notes, process drawings, and video demos.
- Auditory learners benefit from reciting concepts aloud, recording lectures, making rhymes, and speaking through problems.
- Reading and writing learners retain well through handwriting notes, flash card creation, textbook annotation, and journaling.
- Kinesthetic learners remember through tactile aids, role-playing lessons, hands-on 3D models, and active study breaks.
- Blend multiple learning styles for maximal multidimensional engagement.
- Apply tailored techniques to overcome lecture tuning out, test panic, and group project challenges.

In the next chapter, let's double down on building your teen's cognitive strengths with the super productivity power of colour-coding their academic work. Vibrant organizational systems will help with their executive functioning deficits so they can truly thrive at school.

* * *

CHAPTER 6: UTILIZE THE POWER OF COLOR CODING

Your attitude is like a box of crayons that colour your world. Constantly colour your picture gray, and your picture will always be bleak. Try adding some bright colours to the picture, and your picture begins to lighten up. –Allen Klein

How Color Coding Helps

Even if your teen isn't a primarily visual learner, color-coding can still help them get their disorganization under control. When your teens color-coordinate their academic materials, they are leveraging the visual processing strengths many people with ADHD possess (Sinfield, 2014). Color grabs their attention, conveys meaning, categorizes concepts, and infuses their studying with aesthetic intrigue—all cognition benefits!

Let's take a closer look at exactly how color coding will help your teen (Josel, 2023; Sinfield, 2014):

- **Captures attention:** Monotone black-and-white pages can make reading textbooks feel tedious fast. But by using vibrant shades, your teen can keep their concentration honed for much longer through sensory appeal, and this is especially helpful for ADHD minds.
- **Enhances memory:** Teach them to associate a specific color with their learning content; for example, red = math. This makes those associations easier to recall later: "Red things were math formulas." Colors will help your teen cement connections.
- **Categorized content:** They could set up a color-coded system for their different subjects: math is red, blue is for foreign language terms, yellow signals key scientists' names and green is for important literary quotes. Color-coded content will help your teen build some structure around their studying.
- **Provides appeal:** Gazing at an organized rainbow color spectrum feels inherently more satisfying than pages and pages of plain black-on-white text. Their notes will be transformed into pretty collections that make studying almost fun rather than dull drudgery.

So, that's how and why color-coding is going to be a great tool to implement with your teen. Next, let's explore the different classroom applications leveraging colorful ADHD superpowers to strengthen organization, focus, and recall!

Color Code Class Materials

Your teen can start by assigning specific colors to their different academic courses. For example:

Math = Red

English = Blue

History = Orange

Science = Green

Foreign Language = Purple

Then, make sure the supplies that you buy for them adhere to the assigned color schemes. Take a look at the examples below:

- **Textbooks and folders:** Think about covering their math texts in red paper, filing English essays into blue folders, carrying history handouts in orange portfolios, and so on. Visually matching their courses to colors will help to reinforce their connections.
- **Writing tools:** They might use red pens for math, blue pens for English, or orange pens for history. Get them some highlighters, too! Color-coordinated writing and editing styles keep things consistent for them.
- **Flashcards and notes:** Flag their vocabulary notecards purple for foreign language terms. Outline history chapter concepts on orange paper using blue pens for key dates. Colors customize materials per class.

Coordinating their school supplies with their courses by color creates an organized visual environment that constantly reinforces helpful symbolic associations. Keep everything eye-catching and color-coded for a handy reference!

Color Code Concepts

Your teen can even take color coding deeper into their different subjects if they prefer. Some suggestions for this include:

- **Notes rainbow:** They might use various highlighters to color code their class notes—yellow to emphasize key scientists mentioned, green for formulas, blue for theories, or pink for vocabulary terms.
- **Connected concepts:** Another suggestion is to draw idea relationship diagrams that link related concepts together through color-coordinated annotation. For example, they could use red arrows connecting cell parts that interact or blue strings between events triggering psychological disorders.
- **Color legends:** This is potentially the most important tip here for your ADHD teen's busy brain. Make sure they create a color legend to make it clear what each color means across their notes, process drawings, and infographics. Just like map legends translate symbols, they should have a word or a phrase that explains the color-meaning associations in case it slips their mind when studying.

Using colors in this way will help to make their studying process more streamlined.

Apply Beyond School

Clearly, color coordination helps your teen visually organize their schoolwork and studying. However, this technique can aid productivity way beyond their academics, too!

- **Coded calendars:** Your teen could use different color dot stickers to tag their calendar with daily events and organize them by priority level—red for urgent meetings, yellow for important deadlines, and green for routine stuff like practices. This will help them with their independent time-management skills.
- **Household organization:** Label kitchen cabinet shelves or clothing drawer bins with color tags denoting contents—blue for Tupperware, green for mixing bowls, and red for baking sheets. Color-categorized storage will make it easier for them to find and tidy things.

There are infinite possibilities when it comes to using helpful color-coding systems, with benefits that go beyond academia into everyday life. Color coding can help ADHD teens organize their mental clutter externally.

Overcoming Barriers

So, you understand why color-coordinated studying is so intuitively useful. Now, let's go over the practical obstacles that might prevent you from implementing these strategies.

Supply costs: In order for your teen to make use of a

comprehensive color system, they will need notebooks, pens, paper, sticky tabs, and more for each course. For financially limited students, that adds up fast. Here are some ideas for tackling this:

- Ask teachers if certain supplies can stay in the classroom.
- Use online free colouring sites instead of purchasing books.
- Team up with friends and split who buys certain items.
- Use discount retailers, sales, and dollar stores when stocking up.

Seems unnecessary/feeling overwhelmed: After years of struggling academically, an extra effort like colour coding may feel fruitless to some teens. They might also feel overwhelmed by the idea of implementing and managing a whole new study system. Remind them that small changes build momentum!

- Add colour gradually—start simply highlighting class notes.
- Try to help them see it as artistic expression, not extra work.
- Notice and praise their focus and organization improvements, motivating them to expand their efforts over time.
- Request their teacher's help to identify key areas to start colour coding.

Activity 14: Applying Color Coding

Now, take a few minutes with your teen to brainstorm specific ways they can apply colour coding to help organize their academic life. Jot down some ideas below.

Ways I could colour-code:

My English binder:

Studying history concepts:

Math textbooks:

Flashcards:

Class notebooks:

My school locker system:

Don't worry about perfection! Just help them to envision some small, realistic colour-coding elements they can try out. Making the content visually captivating for their ADHD brain could help immensely with their comprehension and recall.

Goal setting:

Based on the ideas you brainstormed together above, choose one or two colour-coding applications to implement this coming week. Write these goals below and make sure you set a date to implement them to help keep them accountable.

I will:

Implemented by [date]:

I will:

Implemented by [date]:

Visualization is the first step toward application. Break it down into doable steps and encourage them to give it a try!

Key Takeaways and What's Next

Let's recap what we covered about the power of colour coding:

- Colour coordination taps into visual processing strengths for those with ADHD.
- Assign signature colours to school subjects and then adhere to schemes across textbooks, notes, and tools.
- Use colours to also categorize concepts within each academic domain.
- Apply colour-coded organization more broadly through coded calendars, household bins, grocery lists, and so on.
- Overcome potential barriers around affordability and skepticism through resource sharing and incremental adoption.

Next, let's see how you can help your teen level up their reading, writing, and communication skills—all of which are essential for academic achievement. We'll explore taking insightful notes during lessons, summarizing key learnings through written reflections, setting progress goals, and developing more literacy skills that will help them achieve school greatness!

* * *

CHAPTER 7: WRITE, WRITE, WRITE!

I can shake off everything as I write; my sorrows disappear, and my courage is reborn. –Anne Frank

Take Great Notes

Try as they might, there is no getting away from note-taking at school. The art of careful note-taking does more than simply capture important lesson details; it also boosts focus, comprehension, and retention of concepts. But a less-is-more selectivity might help your ADHD teen instead of extensive transcribing word-for-word. Below are some top tips for taking great notes you can share with your teen:

- **Prioritize key points:** Encourage them to consider their notes as skeletal frameworks where they can simply identify the main ideas, bolded definitions, numbered steps, and visual sketches. They can leave lower-importance details and examples out and simply summarize lectures efficiently.

- **Leave clarifying gaps:** Note-taking mastery is a skill that develops over time. Initially, your teen will probably leave scattered blank areas where confusion arises, terms need defining better, or examples would clarify the different concepts. They can review their notes again later on and fill in any holes. Eventually, they will deliberately leave gaps that they will intentionally come back to later.
- **Star key content:** Your teen can use highlighter pens, asterisks, and other symbols to prominently tag any essential notes, theories, or takeaways that are going to be most vital for testing their comprehension later.

Thoughtfully concise note-taking amplifies learning. Let's build other reflective writing skills to expand their retention, too!

Summarize Studying

The exercise of paraphrasing what we read and hear helps to solidify new information in our long-term memory (Loma Linda University, 2019). Let's take a look at some tactics you can share with your teen to help them use this to their advantage:

- **Chapter recaps:** Encourage them to pause periodically as they advance through textbook chapters to recap the ideas that have been covered in a paragraph or two. They should identify key theories, sequences of events, cause-and-effect relationships, and overarching themes.
- **Explain in their own words:** Instead of parroting

verbatim definitions from study guides, they should rewrite descriptions of concepts, processes, and systems using simpler phrasing to build their comprehension.

- **Connect to experiences:** They might be able to relate abstract lessons to their own experiences and emotions, which will help them to deepen their resonance. For example, they might link physics friction laws to screeching bike tire skids. Help them to create tangible bonds between their classroom learning and their daily events and experiences.

By regularly synthesizing academic concepts through reflective writing, your teen will be able to build deeper, lasting neural connections.

Journal Reflections

Purchase a notebook for your teen that is dedicated just to academic introspection. Encourage them to spend some time, at least once per week, sitting and writing reflectively about their lessons and learning. They can solidify learning through:

- **Evaluating takeaways:** What resonated with or surprised them about their lectures this week? For example, how might European exploration motives then connect to modern imperialism? Encourage them to probe deeper into the implications of their course material through reflective questioning.
- **Linking to the real world:** Beyond textbook pages, where do the related dynamics of what they are learning unfold in pop culture, current events,

and their personal adventures? Help them to draw lines between classroom concepts and their lived experiences.

- **Considering discussion prompts:** Teachers often pose intriguing perspective prompts like "Would you ever have joined the gold rush?" They could use their journal to imagine, analyze, and defend responses to those hypotheticals. This kind of reflective speculation will help to deepen their comprehension.

Having a set, structured time for journaling will allow your teen to explore more thoughtful reactions, tie-ins, and other questions they might have. Not only will this help them to retain information from their lessons, but it will also teach them how to be reflective and question ideas, which is a skill they can take forward into success beyond the classroom.

Activity 15: Journaling Prompt Sampler

Grab your teen, and let's practice some journal reflection skills! Below are three thought-provoking journal prompts for you to practice with. Take a sheet of paper each and pick one or two of the prompts that intrigue you and your teen. Then, freely write your reactions for five minutes per prompt.

Remember to:

- link classroom concepts to personal experiences
- evaluate information in new contexts
- entertain different perspectives

Prompts:

- How could quadratic equation principles help design fair roller coaster acceleration rates, maximizing the thrill while preventing any whiplash injuries?
- Should high schools teach financial literacy, covering taxes, investments, and managing credit to better prepare teens for adulthood? Defend your perspective.
- If you directed a forest wildlife conservation nonprofit, what actions would you take to balance the preservation of nature while still allowing public access to recreation?

After responding, underline the parts where you:

- related it to relevant life examples
- discussed hypotheticals evaluating an issue
- linked concepts across domains

Once you have both finished, take some time to discuss the process with your teen. Did journaling prompts like these help them to solidify class material while building valuable reasoning skills? How could they use similar idea stimulation to drive engaging studying? Use the space below for any notes you might want to keep here.

Improve Retention

So, how does writing really help? Well, beyond aiding your teen's organization, the cognitive exercises involved in handwriting notes, summarizing concepts verbally, journaling takeaways and mapping goals fundamentally improve learning comprehension and retention (Everson, 2023).

Writing aids memory: Neuroscience reveals that the motor memory incorporated in writing out key bits of information multiple times creates deeper sensory memory than just reading the material (Mathias & von Kriegstein, 2023).

Articulating builds comprehension: Struggling to articulate explanations of processes, interpretations of literature themes, or step-by-step calculations requires deeper mental modelling than passively consuming information really allows. Speaking through the material will help your teen cement their understanding.

So, encourage your teen to wield their pens actively, not just their keyboards! Create accountability around written reflection habits and see if they can take the initiative with this one.

Overcome Writing Obstacles

As we have learned, ADHD minds face executive functioning challenges. These challenges can sabotage their writing efforts, triggering frustrating barriers for your teen. Let's explore the most common obstacles and how your teen can overcome them.

Organizing thoughts: Ideas race chaotically through their minds, arguments lose logical flow, and completing long projects feels overwhelming... help them to reign these thoughts in through:

- concept mapping their first brainstorming associated ideas visually
- outlining their draft structures before composing paragraphs
- setting process-writing goals—not finished products right away

Combating perfectionism: Your teen might be paralyzed while striving for flawless papers or obsess, endlessly starting without ever advancing through their drafts. Remind them that "done" beats "perfect" every day!

- Set tiny word count goals to help them advance through their writing.
- Celebrate their ideas without judging the initial quality.
- Remember, revision refines work, and rough starts are fine! A rough page is much easier to edit than a blank one.

Managing longer papers: Big assignments can be broken down into mini steps to help prevent procrastination and avoidance.

- Encourage your teen to commit to short writing sessions at a time.
- Reward their milestones and efforts instead of reserving praise for the completed project.
- They might even use support groups to establish peer accountability.

While writing can help tap into their strengths, for some students with ADHD, flexibility, compartmentalization, and positivity are really what help them overcome any hurdles and frustrations.

Activity 16: Overcoming Writing Obstacles—Reflection

What writing barriers trip your teen up most often? For this activity, you're going to assess their situation and then strategize solutions together!

Part 1: Writing Obstacles

Check out the most common writing struggles your teen personally faces:

- Perfectionism paralyzes getting words on paper.
- Ideas are disorganized and lacking flow.
- Big assignments overwhelm them, so they procrastinate.
- They are unsure where to even begin.
- They forget key pieces, like citations.
- They are constantly redoing sentences obsessively.
- Something else:

Part 2: Possible Solutions

Given the obstacles identified above, check off two or three solutions that might help boost your teen's writing productivity:

- Set a micro-goal of writing 25 words at a time.
- Try speech-to-text tools.
- Use concept mapping to organize thoughts.

- Establish peer writing check-ins.
- Make citations part of drafting, not after.
- Celebrate ideas without judging initially.
- Something else:

Part 3: Next Writing Steps
Jot down at least two tangible techniques your teen can commit to trying in their next writing session:

Key Takeaways and What's Next

Let's recap what we covered about writing for academic achievement:

- Carefully create lecture notes around key ideas instead of verbatim transcribing.
- Summarize studying through written paragraph recaps and verbal explainers to cement concepts.
- Use the journal to regularly reflect on lessons, tie classroom concepts to life, and discuss hypotheticals.
- Writing and articulating assist memory and comprehension neural pathways.
- Overcome writing barriers through organization tactics, managing perfectionist tendencies, and compartmentalization.

Are you ready to help your teen further flex their mental strengths by setting goals? Prioritization, planning, and realizing their big vision are what come next! Let's help them strategize conquering school, home, and life demands through effective personal development goal planning.

* * *

CHAPTER 8: SETTING GOALS

If you set goals and go after them with all the determination you can muster, your gifts will take you places that will amaze you. –Les Brown

Research shows that setting specific, measurable goals can trigger your reticular activating system—the part of the brain that governs your drive (Arguinchona & Tadi, 2019). Clearly defined goals cause this region to start subconsciously scanning for opportunities to achieve that vision. So, whether your teen wants to boost their math grade or master the guitar, clearly defining their desired outcomes will help kickstart their internal momentum. Goals also provide roadmaps for achieving dreams and help to break your teen's intimidating ambitions into smaller, more doable steps.

Now, let's explore thoughtful goal-setting frameworks to help catapult your teen toward the bright future they envision!

Taking Stock of Dreams

First up, your teen needs to know what it is that they really want in order to set goals in the first place. What do they picture for their future? Do they have an ultimate life vision yet? Encourage them to think about their passions and remind them of their strengths and interests.

If they are struggling with this, turn the discussion to their role models. Who do they aspire to be like? Think about public figures, personal acquaintances, celebrities, and so on. Who do they model their behaviour or their image after? This will help them identify the qualities that they admire and why they want to be like those people.

It might also help to think about what hobbies, activities, or classes keep them effortlessly absorbed for hours at a time. Help them to think about the kinds of things that they are good at and the things that they enjoy and brainstorm ideas for how they can pursue this going forward.

Activity 17: Envisioning Their Best Future Self

In this activity, you're going to let your teen's imagination run wild, dreaming up possible amazing futures for themselves! Set a five-minute timer for them, and encourage them to freely brainstorm responses to the following prompts:

In my wildest dreams for the future, I am a successful

Entrepreneur who:

Performer/artist who:

Activist/leader who:

Teacher/mentor who:

Other career idea:

I admiringly look up to the following people's lives and accomplishments:

My natural talents and interests I could build a purpose around include:

After brain-dumping dream career paths, role model traits, and innate strengths, they should circle two or three options that leap out as most inspiring to them. This activity will give them some idea of what they might like to set their future goals around.

Breaking Down Goal Steps

It's all very well to have a dream or a life goal, but how can you help your teen actually get there?

Set S.M.A.R.T. Goals

This is a skill that your teen can use beyond class-specific learning and something they can use for all kinds of goal-setting in their lives. By using Peter Drucker's S.M.A.R.T. framework, your teen can establish student development goals to build their executive functioning abilities and enable true future success (*What is SMART Goal Setting?* n.d.). Let's look at how S.M.A.R.T. goals work:

S = Specific

Goals like "Do better in math" are much too vague to be practical. Get precise and encourage your teen to set specific goals: "Improve algebra quiz scores from Cs to Bs by studying 30 minutes daily."

M = Measurable

Instead of simply hoping that outcomes will be achieved, help them make their goals measurable so they can track their own progress tangibly. Instead of "Study more often," set a measurable goal like "Study for 30 minutes every evening after school."

A = Achievable

The important point here is to set challenging but *realistic* goals that will stretch their abilities while also ensuring they have the capacity to reach them. Setting the goal to study for 30 minutes every evening after school doesn't work if they have extra-curricular clubs that take up all their free time three nights a week, for example. Help them to set goals that are achievable so they don't feel like a failure the first time their schedule clashes.

R = Relevant

Ensure that there is a link between the goals that they set and their overarching hopes. If they want to go to law school eventually, then putting all their free time into basketball probably isn't the best use of their free time and goal-setting.

T = Time-bound

Deadlines are crucial here; they create accountability by giving them a tangible finish line to aim at, which will help prevent your teen from infinitely delaying their efforts. Commit to action by helping them set concrete calendar due dates for their goals.

Activity 18: Setting S.M.A.R.T. Goals

It's time for your teen to practice applying the S.M.A.R.T. framework to one of their personal goals. Together, select a specific aspiration of theirs that relates to improving an area of their life. This could be cooking more nutritious meals, studying for an hour daily after dinner, avoiding emotional outbursts, journaling daily, or having meaningful conversations with friends every week—anything!

Now, they're going to transform that fuzzy aim into a S.M.A.R.T. goal following these structure criteria:

- **S (Specific):** Precisely define a measurable outcome.
- **M (Measurable):** Quantify how they will tangibly track progress.
- **A (Achievable):** Is the goal realistic yet challenging, given their current abilities? Break a big goal into smaller milestones if needed.
- **R (Relevant):** Explain how this aim ties to a deeper aspiration that motivates them.
- **T (Time-bound):** Assign a start date and a target end date for achieving this goal.

S.M.A.R.T. goal draft:

Review their draft above. Did it meet all S.M.A.R.T. criteria defining a thoughtfully crafted goal? If not, help them to refine it now!

Your teen could share their finished S.M.A.R.T. goal with a peer, too, and get their feedback on whether they think it seems like an effective aim to guide their growth and success.

Staying on Track

Once your teen has some well-structured S.M.A.R.T. goals planned out, the next step is to employ some accountability and celebration systems to keep their momentum flowing toward their goals. You can help your teen by doing some of the following:

- **Post prominently:** Tape their goal statements somewhere visible as a constant reminder and subconscious cue that signals their importance and possibility. Reading those brave ambitions regularly will help to strengthen your teen's resolve when they are tackling daily choices; ultimately, they will align their efforts with their goals.
- **Routine check-ins:** Decide on an appropriate time—whether that be weekly, biweekly, and so on—to spend some time evaluating their progress toward their goals. Have open discussions about their tactics and help them come up with adjustments if needed, or simply pat them on the back for crushing it!

- **Effort rewards:** It's important not to save your praise and rewards for when they achieve the goal itself. Instead, have small celebrations along the way for the consistent effort in which they have invested. Praise them for finishing an outline draft before the final essay is done. Appreciate their effort, not just the milestones reached.

Consistent positive feedback will help keep your teen motivated. They will appreciate your input and ideas for any adjustments they need to make and will glide toward their final goal of achievement, with you cheering them on along the way. Let's now look at how to help them re-evaluate and adjust their goals.

Re-Evaluating and Iterating

Progress isn't always linear, especially for our ADHD teens! It's important to teach them how to be flexible with their goals and be able to respond to challenges and changes over time.

- **Quarterly reviews:** Help your teen build in checkpoints for every academic term or seasonally to fully reassess their goals. During these reviews, they should update their end targets based on their current rate of progress and modify their tactics if certain activities are proving ineffective.

- **Trajectory realignment:** As their dreams begin to crystalize through their new experiences, your teen needs to be able to pivot their goals based on their new interests and strengths. Remind them that growth isn't fixed but emergent.

- **Stretch goals:** To avoid the boredom that might accompany a long-term goal, you can keep them engaged by setting newer, smaller goals that are aligned with their long-term vision.

Repeating the S.M.A.R.T. goal-setting process every so often with your teen will help to make sure their goals are still relevant and that they are still on an upward trajectory, and it will remind them of their long-term vision and why it matters to them.

Activity 19: Quarterly Goal Review

Let's directly apply the practice of reassessing progress and realigning goals as needed! Take some time every three to four months to revisit your teen's long-term goals with them and review them as follows:

Part 1: Celebrate progress!

Look back at 1–2 S.M.A.R.T. goals you set with your teen last term. Identify any components they have successfully achieved so far:

Part 2: Troubleshoot obstacles

Name any parts lagging behind expectations:

Part 3: Iterate tactics

List two or three modified strategies to try this upcoming term to accelerate their desired outcomes:

Part 4: Stretch goals

Given their strengthened capabilities, draft a new, bigger, audacious goal to expand their growth edge:

Setting aside time for reviewing their goals and aspirations will help to prevent stagnation through celebrating wins, adjusting approaches, and continually up-levelling challenges as their skills sharpen.

Applying Beyond Academics

While we've explored S.M.A.R.T. goal setting largely in an academic context here, it's important to note that the framework can be used for self-improvement across all other parts of life, too. Take a moment to consider the following areas of your teen's life and whether setting S.M.A.R.T. goals will help them:

- **Social aims:** Does your teen hope to confidently make new friends, lead youth organization events, or have more meaningful conversations with family and friends? Goal-setting can be used to develop interpersonal skills.
- **Health goals:** Getting fitter, fueling their body with nutritious foods, or improving their sleep consistency—all start by defining specific exercise regimens, meal plans, or sleep schedules. Encourage them to use goal-setting to get serious about their health!
- **Passion projects:** Perhaps your teen has been dreaming of recording an album, publishing poetry

online, or winning a drone robotics competition. They can use the S.M.A.R.T. framework to consider the different checkpoints that will help them meet their bigger vision.

- **Lifetime targets:** Some teens find it impossible and overwhelming to think about attending college, earning an income, or finding housing after they graduate high school. You can help them by setting monthly milestones and letting them take more responsibility for their own lives through goal-setting.

Whatever their aspirations and life goals may be, you can help them scaffold their future by setting S.M.A.R.T. goals now.

Overcoming Barrier Fears

Goal-setting is great for guiding your teen's personal growth; however, deep-rooted struggles like procrastination and perfectionism can seriously undermine their follow-through. Let's take a look at both of these now:

- **Combating procrastination:** Postponing starting tasks is something we *all* struggle with—ADHD or not! The key is to divide bigger goals into daily, digestible, bite-sized objectives. Being able to check those smaller tasks off will give your teen the boost of having tiny, repeated wins, and the "big" goal is no longer so overwhelming.
- **Coping with perfectionism:** Perfectionists endlessly tweak without ever truly finishing a completed

product. Remind your teen that *done* beats *perfect*. Help them to release their expectations of perfection and value consistent effort instead. Celebrate progress over perfection and help them break this barrier.

Activity 20: Goal Obstacles Brainstorm

Let's help your teen assess what factors commonly undermine their goal progress and then help them strategize some solutions! Sit down with them and review this activity:

Part 1: Identify barriers

I tend to procrastinate on goals involving:

____

____

____

Perfectionism paralyzes me when I attempt:

____

____

____

Other obstacles I encounter are:

____

____

____

Part 2: Brainstorm solutions

To combat procrastination, I will try:

____

____

____

To manage perfectionist tendencies, I will:

____

____

____

To address other barriers, I will:

____

____

____

Part 3: Accountability partner

I will ask ______________ to check in weekly as I work toward the goals we set together earlier.

Become your teen's accountability partner and help them identify what potential solutions could help them tackle those sticky goal barriers.

Key Takeaways and What's Next Chapter

Let's go over the different techniques we talked about in this chapter for helping your teen set and achieve goals:

- Encourage them to imagine their big dreams and focus on what they're passionate about.
- Break down their goals using the S.M.A.R.T. framework, setting smaller checkpoints along the way.
- It's also helpful to display their goals visually and regularly check their progress.
- Make sure they keep pushing themselves and don't get too comfortable with their targets.
- Encourage them to apply these techniques not just to school but also to their social life, health, and other important skills.
- Finally, help them beat procrastination by setting small, achievable milestones.

Next up, let's think about the tools at your teen's fingertips that can help them remember obligations and harness their focus—phone apps!

* * *

CHAPTER 9: UTILIZE PHONE APPS

The most effective way to improve productivity is to eliminate work. –William E. Conway, Jr.

You might be thinking that utilizing phone apps sounds like a terrible idea—your teen has been known to endlessly scroll social media feeds or zone out for hours watching clips on their phone. However, it's important to note that their phones *can* be used as a force for good. Let's find out how!

Time Management Apps

Let's be honest: Sometimes, having a diary, a calendar, a notebook, and sticky notes all over the place is not the most efficient way for your teen to manage their time. If they are too disorganized to maintain a written record of their schedule, there are plenty of ADHD-friendly apps that can help them restore order to their minds and keep track of their time and tasks.

Calendars and reminders: Mobile OS platforms like iOS and Android integrate calendars and reminders, allowing your teen to map all of their obligations, assignments, practices, social events, and more in one place for consistent reference. You can even sync these across their devices, so they'll never be caught out.

Task manager apps: Apps like Todoist, Microsoft To-Do, Google Tasks, and more let your teen break down bigger projects into detailed step checklists while prioritizing items. Structuring their work this way will help to break down their progress into smaller achievements.

Habit trackers: Apps like Habitica and Streaks help to establish consistent rhythms around things like exercising daily, practicing instruments, or getting eight hours of sleep. They also visually reward consistency in meeting targets, almost turning it into a game.

Digital time management can be just as effective—if not more so—than keeping a physical record. These apps could be a game-changer for your teen's school success!

Focus Enhancing Apps

Perhaps your teen doesn't struggle so much with their time management; it might be their focus that needs work instead. If that's the case, consider the following digital suggestions for overcoming a lack of focus:

Noise-cancelling: Murmuring crowds or nearby construction can be extremely distracting for the ADHD brain. There are noise-cancelling headphone apps, like

Krisp, that mute environmental sounds so your teen can zero in on work without any random auditory distractions.

Ambient sounds: Some teens actually need more background noise in order to hold onto their illusive focus. Consider soundscape apps like White Noise, which create gentle background audio like raindrops or calm cafes. These background sounds can mask the disruptive sounds around them and help them maintain their concentration.

Website/app blockers: It might also be useful to install apps like Freedom, which restrict your teen from accessing distracting sites like social media for set periods of time. Then, they can mindfully direct their attention to productive workflows without the temptation to drift to social media instead.

Pomodoro timers: The Pomodoro productivity method splits effort into 25-minute intensely focused sprints with 5-minute breaks between to recharge. Apps like Tomato Timer can help your teen optimize this flow, scientifically balancing strain, and recovery for optimal overall output.

The right apps can actually scaffold your teen's concentration and help them stay focused on their studies without the usual distractions preventing them from getting anything done.

Organization Apps

Other struggles for the ADHD teen include organization. Yes, there are tons of ways that your teen's phone can help them with this little setback! Think about the battered notebook currently sitting on their desk; it's been dragged through the mud backward—literally! Consider these digital alternatives to help keep their notes, assignments, and other files organized and tidy:

Note-taking apps: Evernote, OneNote, Google Keep, and more will allow your teen to consolidate their handwritten, typed, and audio notes with tagging and notebooks. This will help them to always find key information fast, even if the original physical copies disappear in the abyss of that locker black hole.

File storage/sharing: Apps like Dropbox, Google Drive, and Microsoft OneDrive offer cloud access to store and securely access files from any device while sharing access with teachers and classmates collaborating on group assignments.

List making and journaling: Consider journaling and list apps to be an external brain where your teen can jot any random to-dos, grocery items, video recommendations, or personally reflective journal entries. These apps bring order to chaos while also serving your teen's self-awareness.

External organizing can be a huge relief for the internal overwhelm in our ADHD teens. Going digital with this can really supercharge their organizing powers.

Memory Boosting Apps

Memory and information retention can be a huge hurdle for those with ADHD. However, as quickly as names, tasks, or deadlines may fly out of your teen's mind, tactical apps can reinforce their retention, counteracting ADHD absentmindedness. Consider the following:

Voice memos: Your teen might benefit from vocally recording reminders, goals, or steps to accomplish. These reminders become like portable, personal pep talks that help them preserve pivotal information that they might otherwise forget.

Flashcard apps: Digital flashcards study platforms like Quizlet and Anki use flashcards, self-quizzes, and other learning tools to help strengthen your teen's memory associations. This can be much more effective than passive revision alone.

Brain training: Games like Lumosity and Elevate involve quick, clever activities that help to train focus, reaction time, memory, and problem-solving skills through addictively fun challenges. These can actually help support your teen's executive functioning skills.

Remembering obligations and critical information can perplex neurodivergent minds. But these apps can help your teen play their way to success and improve their memory.

Learning Assist Apps

Finally, let's take a look at apps that can directly help your teen with their studying struggles:

Dictionaries and calculators: Dictionary apps can help them to decode vocabulary definitions on demand, while math calculators will assist them in solving equations—both handy tools to have on their phones during a study session.

Text-to-speech (TTS) readers: If your teen struggles to stay committed to reading their textbook, TTS apps could be the solution. They convert written content into audio and can help if your teen prefers more auditory-style learning.

Academic apps: From physics formula helpers like Photomath to anatomy 3D visual body atlases like Complete Anatomy, subject-specific apps can help your teen creatively clarify challenging concepts interactively.

These aids are handy for all teens who struggle with studying, not just those with ADHD. Help your teen find their study confidence by investing in some handy, helpful learning assistance apps.

Activity 21: Build Your Teens App Arsenal

Sit down with your teen and take inventory of which apps they currently use to help them—if any! Check off any that they already use, and then write down at least two apps that we listed in the chapter per category that you both think they should try out:

Time management apps

- calendar
- reminders
- tasks/to-do lists
- habit trackers

Apps to try:

Focus enhancement apps

- noise cancellation
- music/sounds
- website blockers
- timers

Apps to try:

Organization apps

- note taking
- file storage
- list making
- journaling

Apps to try:

Memory boosting apps

- voice memos
- flashcards
- brain games

Apps to try:

Encourage them to try out some of the apps they've written down; think about the areas they really struggle in and start there!

Overcoming Tech Traps

Yes, we have spent this whole chapter discussing the benefits and merits of different apps that can help your teen with their studying and executive functioning skills... However... Now, we need to consider the other side of things: distraction and device overuse. As we know, ADHD brains crave neural stimulation (Littman, 2023), so our teens can easily get lost in their devices and struggle with finding balance. What can you do to help?

Avoiding distraction loops: Apps like TikTok or YouTube will inevitably suck your teen's attention span into fruitless hyperfocus wormholes. You can make use of focus app blockers, phone access limits, or parental controls on their phones to prevent them from wasting too much of their study time down random rabbit holes.

Balancing healthy usage: Using apps for schoolwork itself can be a great help; however, excessive recreational screen time can have a negative effect on your teen's vital sleep, physical activity, social connection, and other wellness pillars. Tactically schedule device breaks with them, encourage them to leave their phone downstairs at bedtime, and help them to make plans with their friends rather than spend all their time digitally numbing out.

While apps boost efficacy, it's important not to allow your teen to become reliant on virtual assistants for every problem they encounter. Help them find the balance between real-life practice and relying on apps all the time.

Key Takeaways and What's Next Chapter

Let's recap the top app categories we've uncovered to assist your teen with their ADHD obstacles:

- Calendar, reminder, task, and habit apps create structure in scattered scheduling.
- Noise controls, soundscapes, and website blockers enable distraction-less focusing.
- Note-taking, file sharing, and list apps help them stay organized.
- Voice memos, flashcards, and games creatively cement their memory recall.
- Math helpers, text-to-speech, and academic apps support comprehending concepts.
- But beware of digital dependence affecting their offline wellness!

Up next, let's discover how you can help your teen stay motivated throughout their struggles and school career.

* * *

CHAPTER 10: STAY MOTIVATED

You can motivate by fear, and you can motivate by reward. But both those methods are only temporary. The only lasting thing is self motivation. –Homer Rice

Everything that we have covered here in "Part 2: Schooling With ADHD" has the potential to change your teen's life for the better. The real key, however, is motivation. Before we move on to thinking about home and life with ADHD, let's first explore the key to maintaining motivation for true, lasting change.

Cultivating Curiosity

Certain subjects like math or literature may not instantly engage your teen's focus for hours; however, this is a skill they *can* consciously cultivate. Let's take a look at how:

- **Ask insightful questions:** Mindlessly trying to absorb facts can be a struggle for those with ADHD brains. Teach your teen to try and access a deeper level of learning by asking insightful questions. Perhaps it would help them grasp a math concept if they asked for a real-world example of its use.

- **Explore deeper dives:** Another way to investigate topics further is by encouraging them to dive deeper. They could look into the history of mathematical philosophy or the author's biographies of the texts they are analyzing. Curiosity concerning context will help them expand their interest.
- **Link interests to careers:** Whether they are struggling in a school subject or not, you can help them to stay curious about their learning by linking the topic to their interests and passions, and even go as far as looking into prospective careers that success in each school subject could open up for them.

Guide them at first by asking your own curious questions and showing them how to research a topic in detail. Then, sit back and allow them the independence to explore and discover their own curiosity!

Activity 22: Curiosity Brainstorm

Part 1: Review this list of typically boring school topics. Circle three that tend to make your teen's mind numb:

- grammar/literary analysis
- algebra equations
- cellular biology
- classifying microorganisms
- memorizing historical dates

- styles of art
- astronomy concepts
- economic supply/demand analysis

Part 2: Set a five-minute timer. Challenge your teen to free write, brainstorming a list of fascinating aspects, implications, or questions related to the three snoozer topics they selected that spark intrigue.

Example: Boring topic—memorizing historical dates

- What was daily life like back then?
- How did key events influence modern culture?
- Could we predict future outcomes based on past cycles?

____

____

____

Your teen can use this technique whenever they come across a topic that bores them. It will help them to dive deeper and discover a deeper curiosity.

Sparking Passions

Motivation comes much easier when we're doing something we enjoy or are passionate about. These passions don't have to be centred around school; think about their creative outlets, skills, and hobbies. Get excited with them and let them learn about motivation in a fun and exciting way.

- **Identify energizing activities:** What hobbies effortlessly engage your teen for hours? Gaming, coding, sports, arts, music, writing, crafts, or something else? Encourage them to tap into those talents.

- **Apply strengths creatively:** The skills that they pick up during their most energizing activities can be repurposed. You can guide them to see how their personal hobbies can benefit their academic achievements. Think creatively—perhaps their interest in fantasy gaming will help them craft a story for their English class.
- **Perform passions publicly:** The best part about having a hobby or a passion is sharing it with others. If they're into sports, sign them up for the local team. If they love to sing, check out talent shows. Perhaps they prefer to write, in which case setting them up with a blog will help them reach a wider audience and connect with other writers. Teamwork, encouragement, and the meeting of minds will help them find the skills to self-motivate.

Parents often focus too much on academic skills, forgetting that their teen's outside hobbies and creativity can teach them key motivational skills that can be applied elsewhere.

Overriding Boredom

Boredom can be a huge hurdle, especially when they are already struggling with a busy mind. Study sessions can quickly go off track when homework becomes monotonous and long textbook chapters overwhelm them. Here, it is important to help them inject some variety and community into their study sessions to counteract their disengagement.

- **Multi-modal content:** Sticking to one form of learning can be really tough. Your teen could alternate between reading chapters and watching or listening to conversational videos or audio that explain the concepts. They might also create colourful graphics to accompany their learning, just to break up the risk of boredom.
- **Social studying:** It really helps if your teen can meet with classmates for motivating homework gatherings at cafes, libraries, or at each other's houses. Not only does it relieve boredom, but it also helps to boost memory retention and understanding by discussing concepts with their friends.
- **Incentivizing effort:** Your teen might benefit from using the Pomodoro technique of studying for 25 minutes followed by a 5-minute break—almost like a reward for their short burst of hard work. Or they might find it more of an incentive to have a special treat lined up for when their assignment is complete. Work with them and see how they respond to incentives.

Boredom doesn't have to be a motivation killer if you give them the tools to overcome it!

Combating Distraction

Distraction is another big motivation killer for our ADHD teens; their brains are constantly looking for and sidetracked by different stimuli. What can they do about it?

- **Remove triggers:** If they know they have a big study

session lined up or a looming deadline, encourage them to leave their phone in another room. Remove any other common distractions and find an area with minimal distractions, no household bustle, and where they can get to work.

- **Divided vs. hyperfocus:** Hyperfocus is the most talked-about superpower of the ADHD brain (Saline, 2022). Your teen can avoid their willpower becoming depleted by hyperfocusing fully for short periods of time, working intensely, and then rewarding their effort afterward.
- **Accountability partners:** If they don't want you to be their partner, they might find a friend or a peer who will check in with them regularly. Knowing they are going to be checked up on will help them stay focused and avoid distractions.

You can help to tweak their environment and minimize distractions. Your teen can embrace hyper focusing and add social accountability, and distraction's disruptive power will diminish quickly.

Strengthening Perseverance

Here is where you can shine, parents! Perseverance doesn't come naturally to ADHD teens, who are more aware of their struggles now than when they were kids. Consistent failure can cause teens to give up easily when things start to go wrong as a self-protecting mechanism. This is where you come in—let's explore how you can help teach them this essential skill:

- **Set micro-goals:** Help them break intimidating tasks

down into daily digestible substeps. For example, read five textbook pages instead of the whole chapter at once. These small steps will help them to banish the big picture.

- **Highlight progress:** Visually highlight their progress, whether that be with a satisfying checklist or a colouring tracking graph. Give them credit for every small step in the right direction and recognize each small success.
- **Reward milestones:** Decide together what their rewards should be and then reinforce their efforts that way. They might ask for guilt-free gaming sessions or go out for victory meals after they finish the week's homework—whatever it is, they earned it, so reward them accordingly!

Positive reinforcement is the number-one key to parenting an ADHD teen. Combat the overwhelm and the pressure, help them to move forward in small, incremental steps, and watch their perseverance grow.

Activity 23: Micro Goals Workshop

Here, we will learn how to break down a huge semester project into achievable micro-goals!

Part 1: Draft micro-goals

Identify a semester-long project, passion effort, or major responsibility that your teen needs to tackle. Define three or four specific and measurable micro-goal milestones that they can achieve consistently each week to make consistent progress. For example:

1. Write a one-page outline draft every Monday

2. Complete one chapter of the rough sketch on Tuesdays
3. Finalize the previous chapter on Fridays
4. Research sources on Saturdays

Micro-goals:

1.

2.

3.

4.

Part 2: Review S.M.A.R.T.-ness

Review your teen's defined micro-goals based on the S.M.A.R.T. criteria we explored in Chapter 8: Specific, Measurable, Achievable, Relevant, and Time-bound.

Provide feedback on one micro-goal needing improvement:

Part 3: Tracking and rewards

What weekly progress tracking system and rewards will you implement with your teen to help them stay consistent in pursuing these micro-goals? Discuss ideas with them!

Help them get through their big projects and hurdles by

breaking them down into step-by-step goals.

Key Takeaways and What's Next

Let's recap the key motivation strategies that you've taught your teen in this chapter:

- Ask insightful questions, dive deeper into subjects, and tie them to careers that cultivate curiosity.
- Connect often with inherently enjoyable activities, creatively apply strengths, and share passions publicly.
- Multi-modal content approaches, social peer studying, and milestone rewards override boredom.
- Remove distraction triggers, leverage hyperfocus, and use accountability partners to combat distractions.
- Micro-goals, visible progress tracking, and small milestone celebrations help to build your teen's perseverance.

You've reached the end of "Part 2: Schooling With ADHD." We've covered so much together already, optimizing your teen's school experience with ADHD!

You have discovered how your teen can leverage their executive functioning through goal-setting, planning, and organizing routines. You have maximized their unique learning styles and strengths and customized their study approaches. And most importantly, you have both learned how to stay continually motivated by sparking their curiosity and passions.

Next, in "Part 3: Home and Life With ADHD," we'll explore applying what you've learned in academics so far to help you and your teen conquer home and life demands, too. Discover tactics to help them optimize their emotional regulation, social dynamics, recreation, and self-confidence through ADHD-friendly routines.

* * *

PART 3: HOME AND LIFE WITH ADHD

CHAPTER 11: MANAGING EMOTIONAL DEVELOPMENT/ UNDERSTAND YOUR EMOTIONS

Some of the greatest moments in human history were fueled by emotional intelligence. –Adam Grant

Ever since elementary school, Amelia has painfully stood out from her peers. They all teased her, asking, "Why are you always so crazy hyper?" "If she's not screaming and stomping her feet, she's laughing and pulling silly faces!" They would laugh and poke fun at her uncontrollable mood swings. Even the teachers played a role, constantly dishing out punishments for her silly or disruptive behaviour. Very soon, she began to feel hopelessly rejected and alienated.

Until her parents sought the help of a counsellor, who helped Amelia design a personalized sensory corner in class. They filled it with fidget toys, headphones, and drawing materials for when she needed emotional regulation breaks. The goal was to minimize her disruptive episodes.

As she got older and started high school, she began keeping a feelings journal instead of needing to go to the sensory corner. She would scribble and scribble when she felt herself preparing for an outburst. She began to track her own emotional trends and triggers, and she learned to remove herself from stressful situations before they escalated.

Now that she was beginning to understand herself, Amelia began to befriend other neurodivergent students and bond through their shared struggles and strategies. Amelia also joined the community basketball leagues, which helped her redirect her restless energy. Here, she made even more friends with other interests beyond school.

It had taken her a long time, but Amelia was finally beginning to feel seen and supported. She had made some wonderful friends, learned new emotional regulation techniques, and found her confidence—which had been hiding beneath her misery all these years. Most of all, Amelia found acceptance, not simply from her peers but from herself.

***

So far, you've helped your teen establish such solid skills and systems for conquering their school demands. Now, in Part 3, you'll learn how to help them apply all those same frameworks we built in Part 2—planning, emotional regulation, focus controls, and more—to excel in the home and life domains beyond school.

It starts with understanding your teen's personal emotional experience. Adolescence can be tough for most teens, but for those with ADHD, it can be a really distressing time. Emotional dysregulation can have a negative effect on every aspect of their lives. Let's begin Part 2 by exploring emotional development.

The ADHD Emotional Experience

Teens with ADHD tend to experience emotions more intensely compared to peers (Littman, 2022). This emotional sensitivity surfaces in several ways:

- **Intense feelings and mood swings:** ADHD brains struggle to modulate their reactions. This means that small frustrations can rapidly escalate into emotional explosions. Teens can swing between euphoric highs when everything seems to be going great and then crash into depressive lows during their challenges. They may be unable to self-regulate these emotional rollercoasters.
- **Rejection sensitivity:** We all struggle with the feeling of rejection, but this can be heightened for teens with ADHD. According to Littman (2022), socializing can be tough for these teens; they crave the feeling of belonging amongst their peers and suffer

from higher risks of social disconnection. Therefore, rejection fees are doubly isolating to them.

- **Common triggers and reactions:** As we have learned so far, transitions, goal pursuit failures, academic struggles, social conflicts, and unfamiliar environments are all factors that commonly trigger emotional reactive patterns in ADHD adolescents. They might display behaviours like avoidance, withdrawal, volatile outbursts, or extreme frustration. Your role here is to provide empathy, patience, and external regulation to help counterbalance these big feelings and help your teen eventually build skills themselves.

Developing Self-Awareness

A crucial factor in gaining control over their intense emotions involves increasing your teen's self-understanding. Teach them to notice their physical cues and behavioural patterns that arise during dysregulation.

- **Tune into physical cues:** With the right guidance, your teen will begin to notice their physical sensations like tense muscles, sweaty palms, or a sunk chest feeling whenever they experience anger, shame, or panic. Building their bodily awareness will help them to be aware of an impending outburst, which is the first step in learning how to de-escalate.
- **Identify emotion patterns:** It will help them to keep track of the different types of situations, interactions, or environments that tend to evoke big feelings. Does academic pressure commonly

trigger hopelessness and then withdrawal within them? Does social exclusion enrage them until they progress toward retaliation? Spotting these emotional cycles will help them to develop their self-awareness skills.

- **Journaling:** Encourage them to dedicate notebooks specifically to processing their emotional experiences, jotting down the sequence of triggers, physical changes, reactive behaviours, and the aftereffects of outbursts. Writing will help them to document and put into words the internally chaotic states that they experience. It will give them another perspective on the situation that triggered them while also helping to build their self-regulation through ongoing mindfulness.

Developing emotional intelligence begins by *acknowledging* when physical sensations start to indicate dysfunctional feelings are bubbling up. In this way, it is possible to predict behavioural pattern trajectories based on past incidents and then use journaling to consciously analyze the outburst from a balanced perspective.

Activity 24: Physical Cue Awareness

Let's learn how to help your teen increase their bodily awareness and detect early emotional shifts through physical signals.

Part 1: Common emotions

Check out the sensations below and mark the items that your teen commonly experiences with these reactions:

- frustration

    - tense muscles
    - sweatiness
    - headache
- anxiety
    - nausea
    - trembling
    - fatigue
- embarrassment
    - flushed face
    - stuttering
    - fidgety

Part 2: Sensation brainstorm

Add two more common physical cues that accompany anger, stress, or hurt for your teen:

Anger:

Stress:

Hurt:

Part 3: Reminder tactile aids

With your teen, identify a tactile item that symbolically represents each state that they can touch to help anchor them to the present when they start to feel overwhelmed—this might be a squishy ball for anger, a smooth stone for calm, and so on.

Describe:

The key is recognizing those early bodily signals as they occur and manifest your teen's rising intense emotions. Then, your teen must learn to engage their coping tools to keep calm and in control. Mind-body awareness will help guide their responses instead of their reactions!

Healthy Coping Strategies

When feelings begin to overwhelm your teen, their ADHD brain needs external regulation support to help teach them healthy responses to counterbalance the intensity of those feelings. Introduce your teen to the following techniques and help them find something that aligns with them:

- **Breathing exercises:** Simple, focused inhalation and exhalation techniques will help to prompt physiological calming in your teen. The vagus nerve communicates the sensations that soothe the emotional centers. Guided meditations and utilizing breathing exercises have extended benefits.
- **Talking it out:** Verbal processing can be a huge help when your teen is feeling on the edge of a meltdown. They could come and talk to you, a trusted friend, or a teacher at school, as long as the person listening does so without judgment and can help them talk through their feelings to help them untangle their reactions. Feeling listened to can help extraordinarily.

- **Creative expressions:** Your teen might consider activities such as journaling, music outlets, physical exertion, or arts and crafts projects. These will help them safely channel their bigger emotions into positive manifestations, keeping any brewing escalations in check.
- **Soothing space for self-care:** Having a soothing space for self-care can be a game-changer for the ADHD teen. Create a space with them that is familiar, has soft fabrics, calming fragrances, and their most soothing activities to handbooks if they like to read, or calming music if that is more their thing. This space will help to ground them when they are having a tough time.

Build a go-to coping strategy toolkit with your teen by mixing and matching their favourite, tailored supports. This will help them to regulate their emotions responsively, with better results over time during each dysregulated moment.

Managing Specific Challenges

While those methods can help immensely, let's now take a moment to break down some tactics to help deal with specific dysregulation manifestations of ADHD that our teens may face:

- **Taming anger outbursts:** If your teen is on the explosive end of the scale, you might consider trading their screaming fits for a safe pillow-punching session. This allows them the physical expression that they need without putting anyone else in harm's way. You can always talk about their triggers and feelings later on when they have calmed down.

- **Alleviating anxiety:** You can help them to reframe their anxious thoughts. They might believe that their friends gossiping and laughing without them means that they are judging your teen harshly. Remind them that anxiety thrives on assuming the worst possible scenario. Chat with them and open their minds to other possibilities; perhaps their friends are simply sharing an exciting memory or discussing something silly that happened in a shared class today.
- **Combating shame:** Let's face it, our ADHD teens make more careless mistakes than their neurodivergent counterparts, and this can often leave them trapped in the cycle of shame. Highlight the effort they invested instead of dwelling on any momentary failures. The key is to focus on growth opportunities to optimize their future strategies rather than reserving praise for achievement alone. Remind them that everyone makes mistakes sometimes, despite their best intentions.
- **Handling hurt feelings:** Yep, hurt feelings are going to be a common occurrence, too. Teach your teen that when people are nasty or rude to them, it is more a reflection of the person being mean than of them. Often, people's actions actually reflect their internal, hidden insecurities. Teach them healthy, calming coping mechanisms to help them through these times and give them another perspective to consider, too.

Remember, intense emotions will always pass, no matter how big they are in the moment! Choosing healthy responses through deep breathing, creative diverting, or thoughtful reframing helps your teen build emotional durability by managing distress and disruptions positively.

Activity 25: Creating a Coping Toolbox

Here, you are going to learn how to build literal kits of comforting items and activities that help your teen specifically overcome their emotional chaos.

Part 1: Strategies

Make a personalized list of 6–8 coping mechanisms that could help calm your teen down when they start to feel emotionally overwhelmed. Get creative brainstorming ideas!

Some examples:

- favourite playlist
- glitter jar
- stress ball
- coloring book

My teens list:

-
-
-
-

-
-
-
-

Part 2: Coping kit bin

Time to get crafty with your teen! Using art supplies, physically create or decorate bins that you can use to store these items. Aim for decorations that represent their healthy mental resets. When dry, you can put all the items from their list inside for when they need them.

Key Takeaways and What's Next

Let's recap what we covered regarding handling intense emotions with ADHD:

- Teens with ADHD can have a tough time controlling their emotions, which can lead to big mood swings and outbursts.
- Feeling really sensitive to being left out or having trouble with schoolwork can make things even harder.
- Paying attention to how your body feels when your emotions start to rise can help you find ways to deal with them before they get out of control.
- Talking about what's bothering you, finding fun ways to distract yourself, taking deep breaths or meditating, and finding a cozy, comforting spot can all help you manage your emotions and think clearly

before things get too intense.

- Teens need support from their caregivers, understanding, and help learning how to manage their emotions over time.

Next, we're going to be looking at an idea we discussed earlier: hyperfocus. Let's learn more about this superpower and how your teen can make the most of it to help them in their day-to-day lives.

* * *

CHAPTER 12: UTILIZE HYPERFOCUS

By focusing deeply on just one important thing at a time—hyperfocusing—we become the most productive version of ourselves. –Chris Bailey

The ADHD Hyperfocus Experience

Hyperfocus refers to an intense, sustained concentration and absorption of an activity to the point of tuning out everything else going on around your teen (Flippin, 2023).

This extreme behavioural fixation tends to occur most frequently among those with ADHD on topics that they have an interest in, or that tap into their dopamine-fueled reward motivation (Bhandari, 2022). On one hand, this enjoyable "tunnel vision" can lead to serious, immersive productivity. However, it also carries the risk of neglecting other obligations and losing track of time while they are engrossed in the fixation (Flippin, 2023).

Features of hyperfocus include (Bhandari, 2022):

- enhanced focus capacity
- the ability to see complex details
- elevated performance in the hyperfocus task
- creative flow
- ingeniously problem-solving
- lost awareness of the rest of the world
- lost awareness of bodily needs

While hyperfocus can be an excellent tool for learning and creativity, it can also hinder your teen's flexibility and ability to shift their attention when appropriate to alternative pressing priorities.

There are ways you can help them harness this skill so that it works in their favour instead of against them! Let's first take a look at the common triggers to help you understand and recognize them in your teen.

Common Hyperfocus Triggers

According to ADHD experts, certain conditions are known to trigger prolonged hyperfocus sessions for kids, teens, and adults with attention deficit tendencies (Flippin, 2023):

- **Matching natural interests and talents:** When activities align seamlessly with your teen's innate passions, skills, and strengths, they might be able to tunnel vision intensely for hours. This whole time, they will be absorbed in mastering the task or skill, whatever it is, as their motivation and joy have combined.

- **Receiving positive feedback and praise:** As we've discovered already, positive feedback and praise are excellent tools and motivators for our ADHD teens. This feedback and praise does not necessarily have to be verbal; things like their scores in an online game sitting at the top of the leaderboard and social media likes and comments can also act as positive feedback. The greater the reward, the more they will repeat the hyperfocus behaviour.
- **Competitive environments:** Sports matches and other competitive scenarios can trigger your teen's hyperfocus as well. They may focus only on winning —at all costs! They might dive into training for hours each day. Here, it's the innate cravings for stimulation that drive their relentless refinement of the related skills.

Activity 26: Identifying Hyperfocus Triggers

Here, we will uncover your teen's personal triggers that elicit their maximum concentration capacities!

Part 1: Passions

List three to five talents or interests your teen could eagerly engage with for hours of joyful immersion and easily lose track of time doing:

____

____

____

Part 2: Praise sources

Which of the following sources of positive feedback, recognition, or validation seem to motivate your teen toward repeating their success? Add your own if not listed.

- teachers
- social media likes
- competition leaderboards
- other

Part 3: Competition outlets

Which of these competitive scenarios intensely anchors your teen's focus toward winning?

- debates
- races
- video games
- other:

Now that you know what your teen's triggers are, you will be able to help them channel their hyperfocus strategically in the next activity later in the chapter!

Hyperfocus Pros

You are probably more concerned about the cons of hyperfocus that your teen may already be experiencing. But before we explore those, I want you to fill your mind with all the positives of hyperfocus to show you how wonderful this skill can truly be:

- **Enhanced focus and critical thinking:** Your teen has laser-focused mental precision powers! They might be able to solve complex logic puzzles, computer programming challenges, and other projects that demand layered analysis. All because they have this superpower ability to devote their undivided attention to the subtle details that are missed by most.

- **Elevated execution:** Your teen will likely have the highest level of capability in their hyperfocus topic—whether that's high scores in their computer game or being able to play their musical instrument to perfection. This demonstrates their high level of capability and is a testament to their dedication and motivation.
- **Joyfully immersed:** Hyperfocused hours might feel like mere minutes to your teen who is absorbed in pursuing their talents or interests. They don't lose time in a negative sense but spend hours locked in a joyful state of higher engagement.

Hyperfocus can be a really fulfilling skill for our ADHD teens; it brings them joy and mastery of their personal interests—what a beautiful skill!

Hyperfocus Cons

Unfortunately, intense fixation can carry consequences across your teen's health, relationships, and obligations—you may already be struggling with some of the following (Flippin, 2023):

- **Difficulty shifting into other activities:** As an example, becoming completely engrossed in complex video games can be extremely frustrating for parents and can lead to lots of yelling and arguing at home. Teens might miss dinner, homework, and other planned activities simply because they are so engrossed in their hyperfixation. Not only do they miss other activities, but friction and resentment often arise when they feel forced to move from their hyper-fixation.

- **Obliviousness to bodily needs:** Your teen might find themselves suddenly starving because they are skipping meals for their fixation. They might suffer from dehydration, headaches, and mood swings from a lack of proper nutrition. Hyperfocusing can often lead to neglect of bodily functions.
- **Lost in their own world:** Sometimes, teens can be so fixated on their passion that they seem to lose all connection with the real world. They might spend weeks locked in their bedrooms through the summer break, missing time with their friends and family and losing all track of time and reality.

Like superpowers, hyperfocus holds the potential for both great achievement *and* harm. As we will learn in the rest of this chapter, there are things you and your teen can implement to help them harness this skill and overcome any hurdles associated with it.

Strategically Channel Hyperfocus

Hyperfocus isn't something that you want to squash in your teen. As we have learned, it can be extremely beneficial and rewarding for them. Instead, we're going to learn how to help them strategically channel this and other skills to harness their potential and help them take back control.

- **Negotiate time blocks:** Your teen might be losing their weekends to gaming binges, and you are constantly yelling, arguing, or simply angry at each other all the time. If this sounds like you, try negotiating with your teen and coming up with a structure outlining the free time they have to play *after* they have completed their homework or chores first. Bargaining with your teen will be much more effective than demanding they completely stop their time-wasting passion.
- **Use calendar alerts:** Having a phone is a game changer for ADHD teens. Help them to schedule alarms or calendar alerts that remind them of their priorities so you don't have to. They will be able to take control of their own schedule, and phone alerts will help them to be independent and get their key priorities done.
- **Build general focus skills:** Hyperfocus can be a really useful skill, but you should also help your teen develop general focus skills so they don't rely too heavily on being able to access this technique. They risk inertia and burnout if they believe they cannot work effectively without entering this state. Strong focus skills that they can apply at any time are much more sustainable!

Rather than getting annoyed with your teen about their unpleasant hyperfocus side effects, compassionately build a proactive, collaborative system with them. This will allow them to focus while also handling real-world responsibilities.

Activity 27: Co-Creating a Hyperfocus Plan

Before you start this activity, take a look back at your teen's passions and triggers from the last activity. We are now going to collaborate on designing a personalized system to help your teen leverage their hyperfocus productively!

Passion priorities

My teen's hyperfocus triggers are:

____

____

____

Time block bargains

You are both going to make a commitment now:

Parent: I commit to not shutting down your interests cold turkey.

Teen: I will complete ______ first before diving into marathon gaming, Netflix, or social media sessions.

Calendar alerts

Spend some time with your teen looking over their school, sports, and other activities. Help them plot their schedule into their calendar app and turn on alerts to remind them when to switch activities or take breaks from their fixations. Make sure you check in with your teen to ensure they are adhering to the alerts, but let them take responsibility as much as possible.

Overcoming Hyperfocus Hurdles

Often, finding a balance between hyperfocus and other activities is the real struggle. Hyperfocus can be really useful for building skills and enjoyment, but it absolutely has to balance with real life!

Re-Entry Challenges and Harsh Comedowns

As you probably know already, when an ADHD teen resurfaces after an extended hypnotic hyperfocus session, there can be some emotional dysregulation. Connecting with reality again can be jarring for them, especially when the new obligations require them to be socially flexible—usually, states of hyperfocus are in isolation.

You can help your teen ease this transition. Giving them timed reminders that they are going to have to switch activities is the most effective method. Let them know 30 minutes before they have to stop their activity, then remind them 15 minutes before. After that, alert them every 5 minutes. This will help them adjust to the change and keep control of their emotions in the process.

Balance Hyperfocus and Fun With Other Life Domains

Your teen might believe that they only have fun when they are spending time on their fixations. You can help them explore the joy in other things and balance their wellness in all areas of their lives.

Prioritize self-care, socializing, and physical health. Encourage them to exercise or take a walk, make arrangements with their friends or family, and take time to relax or work on a life skill.

The key here is to teach them about balance and encourage them to spend time attending to all of these aspects of their lives for their overall mental and emotional wellness.

By intentionally honouring all aspects of life beyond their hypnotic passions, we help them to develop sustainable motivation, wellness, and happiness.

Key Takeaways and What's Next

Let's break down how your teen can make the most of their super-strong mental powers that come with ADHD hyperfocus:

- Hyperfocus is when your teen gets really, really into something and forgets about everything else.
- They can use this intense focus by planning specific times to really dive into activities and making sure they balance their responsibilities.
- Setting up digital reminders can help them stay on track and avoid getting sidetracked.
- It's important to help them come back to reality gently after they've been super focused on something.
- It's about helping them stay motivated to grow and develop in different areas, not just the things they're super interested in.

Next, let's learn how to nourish our ADHD teens' minds and spirits by exploring personalized lifestyle design. We are going to be crafting environments and activities that promote harmony. Discover tactical living hacks to reduce restlessness and manage overwhelm through intentional Zen space creation and mindfulness habits.

* * *

CHAPTER 13: YOUR TEENS ACTIVITIES

Design is not just what it looks like and feels like. Design is how it works. –Steve Jobs

As the parent of an ADHD teen, you know the chaos of trying to keep them happy and balanced—we discovered a lot about this in the previous chapter! Some days, they're bouncing off the walls with energy and other days, they'll hyperfocus on Minecraft for hours, completely oblivious to the world around them. Either way, keeping their emotions and energy regulated can feel tricky.

But what if you could design a lifestyle using spaces, activities, and routines that tap into how their unique brains are wired? Instead of always trying to shove square pegs into round holes, the goal is to meet them where they're at.

In this chapter, we'll explore little life hacks you can try at home to set them up for success. Easy things like optimizing their bedroom sanctuary for sleep and creativity and finding physical outlets that let them move —sports, yoga, or dancing to their favourite music video. You might also display inspiring quotes that reinforce their talents, connect with supportive communities that "get it," or simply play games matching their intellectual giftedness.

It's all about embracing the beauty of their neurodiverse brain rather than constantly seeing it as problematic. By tweaking lifestyle factors, you can help them avoid restlessness spiralling into mischief or boredom-breeding anxiety.

Soothing Spaces

Our teens' physical environments can either Zen them out or zap their limited mental reserves faster than a quad-shot latte. You can carefully create a calming space for your teen that builds a serene habitat for their ADHD wiring:

- **Optimize bedroom sanctuary:** Make their bedrooms a cooling, tech-free sleep zone designed specifically for nightly recharging. Modular furniture is great because it allows for adaptable layouts to match their shifting interests and to display their treasured items.
- **Designate calming creative zones:** If you have the space, then carve out an undistracted nook for reading, listening to music, journaling, or other interests. They will quickly come to associate that space with feeling calm and good.

- **Display positive psychology prompts:** You might also consider taping inspiring quotes, hopeful mantras, or courage-bolstering affirmations to their wall or where they will see them often. This will help remind struggling kids of their talents and latent potential yet to be unlocked. Surround them with so much love to boost their self-esteem.

Our homes should be a sanctuary for our teens, not a place of additional hurdles for them to overcome. Let's thoughtfully create havens for them that honour their neurodiverse minds using peaceful organization, inspirational cues, and unconditional understanding.

Activity 28: Soothing Space Vision Board

Building a personal haven aligned with your teen's interests and needs will help bring peace amidst life's storms. Here, we will learn how to craft vision boards to help your teen design their dream sanctuaries that you can then create later on.

Collect

Your teen needs to gather any inspirational images, fabric swatches, colour palettes, quotes, or photos representing their ultimate oasis environment. Consider what brings them joy, calm, and positivity when choosing these.

Ideas:

- favourite colours
- soothing natural elements like water or trees
- cozy textures and lighting features
- uplifting affirmations

- photos of beloved books, arts, pets, or hobbies

Craft

Arrange all of the collected visual elements to create a collaged vision board that showcases their ideal restorative space. They can add descriptive captions, too! Feel free to embellish however they wish; it's important to make it distinctly personal to them.

Create

Now it's your turn to get to work! Now that your teen has designed their ideal space, you can take the time to create it. Include as many elements from their vision board as possible and soak up their joy when they see it for the first time!

Movement

For active ADHD minds, sitting still and studying for endless hours simply fuels their restlessness, and this eventually erupts volcanically—as you probably well know! Exercise and movement can actually help your teen manage their ADHD symptoms as well as make them feel good (Ellis & Seed, 2017). Let's explore their options:

- **Sports matching mobility needs:** High-intensity athletics like basketball, lacrosse, hockey, or even vigorously dancing to their favourite tunes metabolize your teen's excess energies constructively. This really can help hyperactive kids thrive by establishing physical outlets for all that energy.
- **Fun physical hobbies:** More individual pursuits

like karate, rock climbing, hip hop, or skateboarding will teach them to focus while also unleashing pent-up energy. It also builds their bodily confidence and gives them the experience of incremental skill challenges.

- **Mind-body practices like yoga:** Your teen might be interested in gentler physical practices that emphasize mindfulness, breathing, and centring. These are great for teaching your teen to slow down occasionally and counterbalance their busy lives. Schools sometimes even offer free yoga now!

We've all been there—snapping at our teen who just can't sit still. But rather than demanding constant motionlessness, which is exhausting for everyone, encourage them to discover enjoyable, physically engaging pastimes. They will find an outlet for their excess energy while also enjoying a new skill or activity—it's a win-win!

Activity 29: Finding a Movement Outlet

Physical activity can provide the perfect pathway to productively channel all that abundant ADHD energy. Here's how you can help your teen discover the sport for them:

Research

With your teen, search online or ask friends about the different fun options in your local area, like climbing gyms, parkour classes, roller skating clubs, dance studios, or even circus arts schools. What intrigues your teen the most?

List top interests

From that research, write down your teen's top three alluring activity ideas, discovering more:

1.

2.

3.

Schedule trials

Contact those three local options and arrange for your teen to take trial classes; make sure you add the trial times to their calendar or drop them off if it's not within walking distance.

Reflect

After your teen's trials, sit down with them and review what enjoyment levels and flow states arose while they were trying each new activity using the 1–5 scale, with one being the most enjoyable and five being the least:

Activity #1:

1 (most enjoyable)	2	3	4	5 (least enjoyable)

Activity #2:

1 (most enjoyable)	2	3	4	5 (least enjoyable)

Activity #3:

1 (most enjoyable)	2	3	4	5 (least enjoyable)

Which activity was the most fun and fluid for your teen? You can help them schedule twice-weekly sessions for their favourites to help them channel their athletic drive.

Creative Passions

If your teen really isn't sporty and hates the idea of yoga or meditation, then they might benefit from creative passions instead. This can also help them to manage their energy and emotions but in a slightly different way. When creative energy is unleashed, "it increases joy, satisfaction, self-esteem, and motivation" (O'Reilly, 2019). What could your teen take part in?

Arts, Music, and Writing Projects

There are so many options here, from traditional mediums like painting, pottery, and writing poetry to digital options like designing video games, editing drone footage, vlogs, or remixing favourite songs. The appeal here is full creative flexibility. Let's take a closer look at some of the benefits (O'Reilly, 2019):

- **Fluid intelligence:** Pursuing intrinsically motivating making, innovating, and storytelling pastimes helps to build cognitive capabilities like visual-spatial processing, working memory, critical thinking, and reasoning. All of these contribute to your teen excelling in their learning in all domains.
- **Emotional growth:** Whether confidently sharing Japanese anime fan art on Instagram, passionately covering Queen rock ballads, or presenting science

fair exhibits on microbial fungi to judges, public performance pushes creative excellence and boosts their confidence and self-esteem.

There are so many different options that your teen can explore if they have a creative soul. Pursuing these passions will help them develop their intelligence and mental health—not to mention the social side of sharing their work and interests and finding like-minded individuals.

Activity 30: Creative Passion Exploration

If your teen loves to be creative but doesn't have a specific skill they would like to spend time on or develop, you can help them figure this out with this activity.

Catalogue their current creative pursuits.

What existing artsy endeavours currently captivate your teen so much that they lose track of time while being immersed joyfully? Photography? Guitar covers? Haiku poems? List their current creative outlets below:

-
-
-
-
-
-

Set S.M.A.R.T. artistic goals.

Form one or two S.M.A.R.T. goals around attempting new creative mediums and applying strengths uniquely

—for example, Publish three nature iPhone photos to Instagram weekly. Don't forget to include deadlines!

(Remember the S.M.A.R.T. framework: specific, measurable, achievable, relevant, and time-bound)

Track new avenue progress.

Help your teen track their progress by reviewing their goals, timelines, and new skills. Motivate them to keep practicing and watch as their creative skills blossom!

Intellectual Pursuits

Gifted ADHD minds often thrive when faced with intellectual challenges. They can tap into their innate strengths and fascinations—especially when there is a little friendly competition involved! If your teen is interested in more intellectual pursuits, consider the following:

- **Games nurture giftedness:** Games and simulation projects allow your teen to display their natural brilliance through teamwork. Consider activities like Scrabble (they can even play online!) and coding camps.
- **Academic interest clubs:** Every passion, from astronomy to zoology, will have its own clubs and circles where your teen can go and meet like-minded individuals. They can share their interests and grow their perspective by seeking kindred spirits.
- **Niche expertise mentorships:** If they have a real niche

interest, you might consider researching places where they could find a mentor, enroll in an intern scheme, or shadow a professional to help them learn more about their career options.

You can cultivate your teen's intellectual skills and interests by helping them find and bond with like-minded communities. This will help them build their confidence and capabilities, potentially even leading them into a future career!

Social Connections

All humans require meaningful social connections for our well-being. Making social connections isn't always easy, however. Perhaps you could encourage your teen to take part in kind community service. Volunteer opportunities like animal shelters, community gardens, and peer tutoring will help them build empathy and leadership skills, as well as meet others and make friends. At the same time, they get to support causes bigger than themselves.

For ADHD teens, it can be helpful to find thoughtful niche communities, as these can provide particular validation, encouragement, and, most importantly, understanding. Encourage them to join support groups where they can share their struggles and strengths. Online and local meetups are available out there. Your teen can learn and share their ADHD life hacks, find motivation, and find a sense of camaraderie, all of which makes handling their ADHD hardship more hopeful as they realize they're not alone.

Besides finding external social opportunities, you can

help your teen make time for quality time with friends and family. Schedule consistent, device-free hangouts where you play their favourite board games and trade life updates during lingering meals. They might even simply go walking for ice cream with their cousins or friends while venting their frustrations and building their bonds.

Having a strong social network will help your teen feel accepted and important. They will be motivated and have the support of their loved ones through the good and the bad times.

Key Takeaways and What's Next

Let's go over the important lifestyle tips we've talked about in this chapter that can really make a difference for teens with ADHD:

- We've learned how to set up our teens' spaces to help them feel calm and focused.
- Giving them opportunities to move around can really help them concentrate better.
- If they're not into physical activity, encouraging their creative interests can also make a big difference.
- Building a supportive community for them and helping friends and family understand their needs is key.

It's important to remember that when teens with ADHD are bored or restless, they can feel really frustrated. But by creating the right environment for them, we can help them reach their full potential.

Next up, we'll be navigating those infamous

social struggles many neurodivergent teens face, like forging and maintaining friendships through enhanced communication.

* * *

CHAPTER 14: SOCIAL DEVELOPMENT/ INTERACTING WITH OTHERS

A good life depends on the strength of our relationships with family, friends, neighbours, colleagues and strangers. –David Lammy

Relationships rock when they are mutually uplifting. However, for ADHD teens, their neural wiring and mood instability can mean that they struggle with socializing and maintaining friendships (*ADHD in Social Situations,* n.d.). If you find that your teen is feeling increasingly lonely, then you are not alone!

In this chapter, we will unlock techniques to help your teen enhance their communication skills, build friendships, overcome conflict, and boost their teamwork.

Enhancing Communication

In their communication, some of the things your teen might struggle with include (Wheeler, 2023):

- interrupting
- talking too much
- going off-topic
- forgetfulness
- finding the right words
- missing the subtext
- impulsivity
- distractions
- long conversations

In order to help them overcome these challenges, there are some skills you can work on with your teen:

- **Active listening tactics:** Active listening means listening beyond the words that are being spoken to truly understand what is being said (Cuncic, 2022). Teach your teen to connect by committing to the following:
    - intentionally focusing on what's being shared without interruption
    - asking curious, clarifying questions
    - summarizing takeaways and showing genuine

understanding

- **Non-verbal cues reading/mirroring:** Encourage your teen to look for gestures, facial expressions, and body language that might hint at the speaker's true emotions beneath the words spoken. They can also reflect body language that displays engaged empathy, letting the speaker know they are being heard.
- **Conversation etiquette skills:** You can role-play with your teen to help them grasp specific conversation skills. Things like:
  - taking turns
  - allowing pauses before responding
  - covering their mouth if coughing or yawning mid-chat

Up next, let's help your teen revolutionize their relationships by practicing their verbal and non-verbal listening skills!

Activity 31: Communication Upgrade Role-Plays
Part 1: Active listening

This is a great activity that you can do with your teen to help them practice this key communication skill. Let your teen be the speaker first so you can demonstrate the kinds of things they should be doing, and you will be the listener.

The speaker will share a two-minute personal story while the listener practices tactics like eye contact, paraphrasing, and summarizing emotional takeaways.

Next, reverse roles and let your teen have a go at active

listening. Give them real-time feedback after the session. You can return to this activity again and again to help them practice this key skill.

Part 2: Non-verbal mirroring

This time, sit facing each other and mirror each other's body language exactly—smile when they smile, furrow brows simultaneously, and so on while you are chatting. Afterward, discuss how the body language shifts helped to deepen the conversation.

Part 3: Etiquette upgrades

Now, you can demonstrate polished etiquette and politeness together by respectfully allowing pauses before interjecting, covering coughs politely, and other scenarios acting out. If you have noticed something that your teen persistently struggles with in conversation, this is a good time to kindly coach them through it.

Part 4: Insights and Applications

Make time after the activity to discuss the kinds of communication upgrades that your teen would like to implement moving forward from these role-play insights. Help hold them accountable for this commitment by practicing with them regularly!

True understanding only surfaces through ongoing practice and demonstration, so it's important for you to do this activity as often as your teen needs. They should commit to applying the communication skills they have learned here in their real-world encounters, and soon, they will notice they are having stronger and more successful conversations.

Building Friendships and Relationships

Friendships are so important to help your teen feel a sense of belonging and support. Having friends will also boost their overall happiness and reduce their stress (Mayo Clinic Staff, 2022). True, enduring friendships that stand the test of time rely on sharing vulnerable spaces, reliable accountability, and loads of compassion. Let's explore some tips to share with your teen that will help them foster great friendships:

- **Expressing empathy and compassion:** Encourage your teen to check in with their friends often. This ensures that any friends facing failures and hard times feel respected and heard. Sharing problems with friends normalizes the reality that everyone makes mistakes and that their efforts are what's important.
- **Responsible reliability in supporting friends:** If your teen can keep their commitments to their friends, this will help to create trust. These commitments might be promised homework-help sessions, attending their tennis matches, or even keeping secrets. Consistency, reliability, and trust are important elements of every friendship.
- **Creating safe vulnerability spaces:** Teens often face judgment and criticism wherever they go. If your teen can foster an environment where both parties can share celebrations, insecurities, family dynamics, or other intimate topics without judgment, their friendships will deepen over time.

Meeting other teens isn't the problem, but building lasting friendships really can be a struggle for our ADHD teens. Share these tips with them, and they will begin to build friendships that will last for decades.

Romantic Relationships

It might be strange to think about your teen having romantic relationships, but it will probably happen sooner than you were expecting. You can play a vital role in helping them prepare for this exciting time in their lives. Whether they come to you with a relationship question or you want to help get them ready in advance, consider teaching them the following tips and skills:

- **Setting healthy boundaries:** Teach your teen to openly discuss and establish mutually enjoyable activities, pet name preferences, and other boundaries early on. The healthiest partnerships are built on a secure attachment where both people feel respected.
- **Direct communication about needs:** Encourage your teen to communicate their needs clearly. These might be centred around the pace of intimacy, needing frequent words of affirmation, or quality one-on-one bonding time free from digital distractions. Everyone has different preferences, but nobody is a mind reader—teach them how to verbalize their needs early on to prevent future relationship problems.
- **Embracing differences lovingly:** Your teen might be concerned that their ADHD symptoms like forgetfulness, hyper-focusing on niche interests, or chatterbox enthusiasm may irritate their partners

over time. You can show them that embracing each other's perfectly imperfect humanness with compassion builds strong foundations for the long run. Their future partner isn't going to be perfect either!

Overcoming Conflict

Fighting with friends or family happens to the best of us. When you're an emotionally dysregulated ADHD teen, it might happen more often. Here is where you must teach your teen that how we handle disagreements makes all the difference between strengthening bonds and damaging trust. Let's do some practical work to teach your teen about staying cool through conflict and not escalating or cracking under pressure!

Know Your Triggers

When someone's comment makes your teen's blood boil instantly, that's a trigger situation. Encourage your teen to pay attention to what exact words or actions tend to set them off, and then they can strategize techniques for self-calming before they react badly.

Activity 32: Conflict Triggers Tracker

Instructions: For one month, your teen should record three situations that caused them frustration or anger, along with the specific reactions that got sparked. Identify the trigger words, actions, or scenarios involved. They should also note down their responses and reactions.

For example:

Week one triggers:

1. My Brother teased me as a "fraidy cat" = Yelled insults

Week one triggers:	How I reacted:
1.	
2.	
3.	
Week two triggers:	How I reacted:
1.	
2.	
3.	
Week three triggers:	How I reacted:
1.	
2.	
3.	

After the month's review, sit with your teen and complete the following:

- Highlight their most common triggers across the four weeks.
- Circle the reactive responses that they regret and want to improve.
- List healthier coping tactics they can try next time those triggers arise again, like walking away or communicating hurt feelings respectfully. Use the

space below to list out some suggested coping tactics:

Take Chill Out Breaks

Before a shouting match about misunderstandings goes too far, teach your teen to call for a timeout. If they are prone to explosive outbursts, they should walk away to chill out and calm down before approaching the situation again. Encourage them to put some space between the frustration and their reaction. This does not mean escaping conflict but giving their head some solid thinking space.

Activity 33: Cool-Off Strategy Brainstorm

List at least two healthy or calming places or activities where your teen can take mini timeouts to decompress when they are upset. This will help keep them from reacting poorly:

1.

2.

Use "I Feel" Statements

During conflict, it is so easy to start blaming and accusing. Instead of hurtful blame games, your teen can share their own feelings vulnerably. Teach them to say, "I feel betrayed when I'm not invited to hang out," rather than, "You backstab me when you exclude me!" Using "I feel" statements will help stop the conflict from becoming a shouting and blame match and pave the way for making simple, respectful requests to reconcile—no demands and no name-calling!

Activity 34: "I Feel" Practice Session

Using "I feel" statements allows for calmly sharing hurt feelings or needs without attacking others. Let's practice with your teen!

With your teen, take turns pretending the other person has wronged you in some way and script "I feel" statements about it.

For example:

- "I feel frustrated when my music is played without permission."
- "I feel rushed when you tell me to get ready for school."
- "I feel annoyed when you leave your dirty laundry on the bedroom floor."
- "I feel left out when you take my sister for ice cream without me."

You can end the activity by role-playing how to reconcile respectfully.

What other conflict-coping tactics have helped you stay cool when tensions run high? You can share these ideas with your teen and discuss other ways they might resolve conflict. The goal isn't pretending there isn't a problem but hashing things out gently yet assertively. Stuffing anger down just delays conflict. Help them to navigate these scenarios maturely and effectively.

Boosting Teamwork

Your teen is going to encounter lots of teamwork

opportunities and requirements throughout their life and school career—whether it's through collaborative school projects, sports teams, or community service groups. Those with ADHD may struggle with teamwork due to things like (ADDA Editorial Team, 2023):

- tendency to procrastinate
- disorganization
- poor planning skills
- poor time management

Teamwork can be really challenging for our ADHD teens, but certain tricks can help.

- **Understanding various roles:** Make sure your teen understands that everyone has strengths on a project. It can be helpful to map out who has what role in a group project. Making a note of each contributor's strengths can help them divide up tasks suited to what people are naturally good at.
- **Mutual understanding and compromise:** When ideas clash around who is the "leader," or if there are any misunderstandings preventing progress, your teen can use some of the communication skills they have learned so far to help find a compromise. Everyone on the team should feel respected, heard, and on board. Encourage them to avoid headbutting and focus on moving forward!
- **Celebrating diverse contributions:** Encourage your teen to openly praise their teammate's strengths, which will help to lift team morale. Whether they are wrangling supplies, telling perfect jokes when

frustrations run high, or teaching everyone cool new digital editing skills, your teen knows that validation and praise matter!

Key Takeaways and What's Next

Let's recap the skills that will help your teen enrich their relationships with friends and partners alike:

- Improve communication by really listening, understanding body language, and being polite.
- Build trust by being reliable, open about feelings, and showing kindness.
- Learn how to set healthy boundaries in romantic relationships and talk openly about intimacy.
- Deal with conflicts in a mature way by staying calm, finding compromises, and expressing needs calmly.
- Understand different roles in a group, be flexible, and appreciate everyone's strengths.

Next, let's build confidence and self-assurance from the inside out. We're going to take a deeper look at building your teen's self-esteem! The goal is to appreciate neurodivergence as an asset, not a hindrance!

* * *

CHAPTER 15: SELF-ESTEEM

Love yourself first, and everything else falls into line. You really have to love yourself to get anything done in this world. –Lucille Ball

As a parent, there are very few things that hurt more than when you hear your child say, "What's wrong with me?" or "Why am I always in trouble?" When ADHD symptoms like poor focus, hyperactivity, and impulsiveness persistently bring about criticism, disciplinary action, and peer rejection, kids will internalize the constant negativity. This might then erode their self-esteem over time (Sreenivas, 2023).

You can help safeguard your teen from that shame, depression, or worse by taking proactive steps to help them build confidence and self-worth early on. This chapter will equip you with the necessary skills to nurture their innate strengths through consistent praise, framing their struggles compassionately, and reassuring them. They are so much more than their limiting labels!

Identify Your Teen's Strengths

It's so easy to get stuck on all the things our ADHD teens need help with or struggle with. In order to help them build their own self-esteem, you should be their biggest cheerleader by highlighting their strengths and encouraging them to do the same.

Pinpoint Passions

What specific activities completely hook their attention for hours? Is it filmmaking, coding video games, or even playing guitar? Watch them and help them figure out what their passions and talents really are.

Activity 35: Superpowers Brainstorm

Sit with your teen, and together, make a list of three activities or skills they can immerse in for hours, losing all track of time.

1.

2.

3.

Next, brainstorm how they could spend more time cultivating these passions. Perhaps they need more supplies if they are arty and crafty, which is where you come in as you can help them gather the things they need. If they need to carve out more time for their guitar practice, help them look at their schedule to see where they can fit it in. Remember, this is a team effort. The more you notice their strengths, the more they will, too, and this will boost their self-esteem.

List Little Wins

Unfortunately, kids internalize criticism more easily than praise. The negative messages they receive can cause them serious problems with their self-image. You can help them by intentionally logging examples of your teen's progress, intelligence, and kindness in an ongoing journal. They can look back on these positive notes when they are feeling down.

Activity 36: Kindness Jar

A cute idea for boosting your teen's self-esteem and confidence is to create a kindness jar. Every time you see them doing something kind, helpful, or wonderful, write it down on a scrap of paper, scrunch it up, and add it to the jar. Eventually, there will be a full jar of kind deeds, and when your teen is feeling low, they can pick a random note out and get a confidence boost.

Ask Others What They See

It can be really helpful for your teen to get an outside perspective on their strengths. After all, you're their parent; you have to tell them how wonderful they are! Encourage them to ask around for positive feedback from teachers, relatives, or family friends, highlighting the kind qualities they see in your kid. They might say things like mad soccer skills or excellent writing. This can really help ease any distorted views your teen has of themselves.

Activity 37: Compliments Survey

Encourage your teen to ask three family members what

positive qualities they admire in them, then note the similarities between the qualities. This will help them figure out what their core strengths are.

Bonus idea: You can even print and frame their favourite compliments and display them like affirmations in their bedroom!

Overcome Negative Self-Talk

Self-talk is something we all do, and it is often linked to past experiences, core beliefs, and distorted cognitive processes (*7 Ways to Combat Negative Self-Talk*, 2018). This is why our ADHD teens might be more likely to struggle with it. If they are constantly criticizing themselves, this negative self-talk will drag down their self-esteem and sabotage their chance at success. Let's develop tactics for quieting cruel inner voices.

Flip Criticisms

With your help, your teen can deliberately reframe their negative thoughts. For example, getting a C in math doesn't mean they are stupid; it means they have to study more. Every negative thought can be flipped like this if you give them tools.

Activity 38: Self-Criticism Makeover

In the space below, write out some of your teen's negative thoughts and guide them in reframing them into a lesson:

Negative thought	**Reframed**
e.g., My room is always a mess. I'm so	I struggle with executive functioning. I can put the

disorganized.	planning and organization skills I learned earlier in the book into practice.

Interrupt Spiraling Thoughts

Does your teen tend to focus on the negativity and then spiral out of control into a void of depression? If that sounds like your teen, don't worry; there are some techniques you can teach them to help!

Instead of spiralling down that negative path, encourage your teen to redirect their attention to gratitude or their accomplishments with the following techniques (*7 Ways to Combat Negative Self-Talk*, 2018):

- Teach them to visualize pressing pause on a remote when their thoughts start getting away from them. Then, they can imagine they are switching channels.
- Ask your teen to name three things that they are grateful for when they seem to be spiralling. They don't have to be huge, revolutionary ideas; simply being grateful for their coat on a rainy day is enough to disrupt negative thought patterns.
- Sometimes, simply talking about their negative thoughts with someone they can trust will help immensely. Help them identify two or three people they can go to when they start to get lost in

negativity.

See Mistakes as Growth Lessons

When your teen is feeling like they are suffocating from the weight of their mistakes, help them to look back over their past mistakes. They've had hard times before, and they certainly will again—remind them of how far they have come.

Activity 39: Growth Mindset Journaling

In the space below, help your teen jot down mistakes they have made in the past and also identify the lesson they learned from it. Use the following table:

Mistake made	Lesson learned or achieved since
e.g., failed English exam	I planned in study time, and now I am averaging a B

If these techniques aren't helping, they can always seek out professional help, and they might find relief through cognitive behavioural therapy (*7 Ways to Combat Negative Self-Talk*, 2018). Negative self-talk doesn't have to rule your teen's life!

Boost Self-Image

Being a teen is tough, especially when it comes to self-image. These days, they have to face endless criticism and ideals splashed across social media, and most of it makes them feel unworthy! That's not to mention the fact that teens are experiencing the biggest physical changes of their lives so far. Here are some tips for helping your teen boost their self-image:

- **Focus on character overlooks:** At the end of the day, personality, passions, and principles outlast superficial stuff. So, encourage your teen to read inspiring role-model biographies in beauty magazines. Get them to follow activists on social media, not just influencers. Point out their good qualities that have nothing to do with looks: Are they kind, helpful, or empathetic? Who they are matters more than what they look like. If you focus on character overlooks, then they will follow your lead.
- **Surround them with body peace:** What they see and are exposed to on a daily basis will inform their idea of what looks good and what doesn't. If they are constantly comparing themselves to an influencer on social media and complaining about how they can't keep up, it might be time to unfollow that person. Introduce them to influencers who are embracing their normal figures and coaches who focus more on self-love than making unhealthy and unrealistic comparisons.
- **Avoid playing the comparison game:** Instead of envying others, redirect your teen to appreciate things about them that are unrelated to their looks. If your teen complains that Isla's makeup is always perfect and theirs isn't, point out the other strengths

that Isla has. "She was also so confident in the school play, wasn't she?" Help your teen see beyond the physical comparisons. Life is not a competition; teach them to see the beauty in everything—not just the physical!

Activity 40: Crafting Self-Esteem Affirmations

As we have learned in this chapter, words shape the inner worlds of our teens. They can either nurture their confidence or slowly corrode their comfort within their own skin. Affirmations are a wonderful way to remind your teen that they are worthy each and every day.

Let's help them craft some compassionate daily affirmations that will help them to reflect their best selves back lovingly.

Part 1: Core values brainstorm

Quickly list three to five words that capture the virtues that are most important to who your teen is deep down. For example, are they creative, loyal, or determined?

1.

2.

3.

4.

5.

Part 2: Strengths shout-outs

Next, note down any strengths and talents your teen possesses that make them uniquely awesome. For example, humour, team spirit, or musicality.

-
-
-
-
-

Use the notes that you have made above as inspiration. You are now going to create four personalized affirmations with your teen that they can read aloud every day to boost their self-esteem. Make them specific and personal by using the "I..." language.

- I boldly express my ____________________ pursuing my passions despite fears of failure.
- I shine by ______________________, spreading more joy in the world.
- I _______________________ facing all the challenges life brings courageously.
- I ______________________, and that makes me amazing just as I am.

You can tape these loving mantras near their bathroom mirror or by their bedsides, as long as it is somewhere they will see it regularly.

Key Takeaways and What's Next

Before moving on to our final chapter, let's quickly recap the core lessons we have covered here for boosting self-esteem:

- Acknowledge your teen's natural talents and keep a record of their daily victories to build confidence.
- Help them to shut down those negative inner voices and shift their perspective to a more positive outlook.
- Encourage them to embrace their mistakes as opportunities for growth and building long-term resilience.
- Focus on developing their character rather than getting caught up in superficial appearances.
- Curate their social media to celebrate realistic beauty standards and positive body image.

Loving yourself might sound simple, but it's incredibly powerful for your teen's mental well-being and success. Next, we'll focus on nurturing their optimism and resilience to tackle external challenges beyond their control while keeping their inner light shining bright.

✻ ✻ ✻

CHAPTER 16: KNOW YOURSELF BETTER, BUILD YOUR CONFIDENCE, AND BELIEVE IN YOURSELF

> *Believe in yourself! Have faith in your abilities! Without a humble but reasonable confidence in your own powers, you cannot be successful or happy. –Norman Vincent Peale*

In this final chapter, you and your teen are going to learn how to embrace their unique ADHD self—all of their quirks, skills, creativity, and general wonderfulness!

Help Your Teens to Know Themselves Better

ADHD minds thrive differently from neurotypical ones.

As you have navigated this book together, you have come to learn how wonderful that really is. You have discovered their superpowers, their strengths, and their battles with their unique struggles. Helping your teen to know themselves better involves simply acknowledging, understanding, and embracing their differences.

- **Understand how their mind is wired:** ADHD brains crave constant stimulation and novelty. But this also often comes with the ability to hyperfocus and do great things (Littman, 2017). Your teen is capable of harnessing all the strengths they have discovered during this workbook now that they have a better understanding of *why* they behave the way they do and *how* to train their unique brain.
- **Appreciate how ADHD gifts them:** Instead of the frustration and limitations your teen used to have around their ADHD, they have now discovered that their restless creativity brews fresh ideas and bypasses conventional wisdom. They no longer see their diagnosis as a hindrance but as a gift that they can use to overcome their struggles. Their operating systems are different, not damaged.
- **Reflect on how ADHD manifests for your teen:** Beyond their general ADHD traits, your teen is now equipped with a personalized understanding of their concentration, emotional regulation, and organization. Through the workbook activities, they have discovered their strengths and weaknesses and uncovered strategies to help them navigate their diagnosis.

Activity 41: Your Teen's ADHD Profile

In order to help your teen know and understand themselves better, let's take the time to map out their unique ADHD strengths, growing edges, and customized supports that they have discovered throughout this workbook. We're going to consolidate them all here in one place, and this will help set them up with everything they need for success!

Reflect back through the workbook to help you fill in your teen's unique ADHD profile.

My ADHD superpowers

I hyperfocus easily when:

My creative strengths shine through:

My ADHD kryptonite

I struggle to stay focused on the following:

Distractions derail me like:

My most disorganized spaces are:

My custom supports

Accommodations that would help me thrive include:

Activities matching my strengths to try are:

I am wonderful because:

Build Their Confidence

We learned in the previous chapter that the constant negative messaging that our ADHD teens receive in their lives can be devastating to their self-esteem (Sreenivas, 2021). We discovered how to help them overcome negative self-talk and boost their self-image. Here, we will discover some ways that you can help them build their confidence:

Challenge Comfort Zones Step by Step

Encourage your teen to try out things that seem a bit scary to them but that are also exciting, like making friends with outgoing classmates, trying out for a play, or giving aerial silks gymnastics a shot—or any other kind of sport they're interested in! They can start by taking small steps to build their confidence rather than diving in all at once. Each tiny step beyond their comfort zone is a win!

Activity 42: Bold Bucket List

Spend some time brainstorming with your teen. See if you can come up with five activities outside of their current comfort zone and capabilities. For example, make friends with a new neighbour, join the football team, or try ice skating.

1.

2.

3.

4.

5.

Now, choose one and break it down into small steps so it doesn't feel so overwhelming. Help them schedule these activities in their lives.

For example: Make friends with the new neighbour.

1. Introduce myself by giving them a "welcome to the neighbourhood" gift.
2. Offer to show them around the neighbourhood or the school.
3. Invite them out for pizza one evening.

Use this space to help your teen step out of their comfort zone:

1.

2.

3.

4.

5.

List Small Daily Acts of Bravery

Confidence isn't something that miraculously develops overnight; it's something you and your teen will have to work on over time. You can help them by noticing and pointing out every time they display an act of bravery or do something outside of their comfort zone. For example, if your teen hates speaking on the phone, praise them for answering a call and overcoming their fear.

With persistence and hard work, you can help your teen develop their confidence skills.

Help Your Teen Believe In Their Potential

The greatest thing you can do as a parent is to role-model the kind of behaviour that you want to foster in your ADHD teen. If you believe in yourself and you believe in others, then they will, too!

Here are some tips to help them see what they are capable of:

Activity 43: Visualize Your Ideal Future Self

Grab a bunch of magazines and flip through them with your teen. You are looking for pictures that represent your ultimate dream job. Maybe it's being a cool DJ, a tech genius creating the next big thing, or a caring nurse making a difference in people's lives.

Next, cut out those pictures and create a vision board, like a collage, that you can put up where they'll see it every day. It's like a visual reminder of their dreams, even if they seem far-fetched right now. But seeing those images every day can inspire your teen to take focused action to make those dreams a reality. It's a fun and creative way to keep their goals in sight and stay motivated!

Activity 44: Look Back at Progress Made

Help your teen tackle those pesky "I'm never getting better" thoughts head-on. Encourage them to look back and take note of all the progress they've made already.

Do they remember those disastrous muffins they used to bake? Now, they're whipping up Pinterest-perfect recipes! And those messy, disorganized essays? They've transformed into solid A grades. Your teen's journey may look slightly different, but reminding them of where they have been and how they have improved in different areas can really motivate them going forward. They've already come so far! Celebrate that with them and encourage them to keep believing in themselves because they are amazing!

Activity 44: Affirm Dreams Daily

You are going to be crafting affirmations with your teen in this activity. Start by writing down at least three bold "I am" statements that declare your teen's victories as if they've already come true:

e.g.:

I am... heading to my dream college to study law

I am

I am

I am

Then, encourage them to say them out loud and record them on their phone so they can listen to their affirmations whenever they need a pick-me-up. It's all about using their imagination to bring their dreams to life and set themselves on a path to success.

This is a great way to stay focused and positive as they work toward their goals! When your teen really believes in themselves, that's when they become an unstoppable force.

Key Takeaways

In this chapter, you have uncovered ways to help your teen feel super confident and believe in their potential. By now, your teen will be able to do the following:

- Embrace their unique strengths and appreciate how your brain is wired.
- Identify their natural talents and create the right conditions to make the most of them.
- See mistakes as opportunities to learn and improve and face their small fears consistently.
- Develop a positive mindset by visualizing their goals, celebrating progress, and speaking affirmations

about their dreams.

Remember, they've got what it takes to handle life's ups and downs with courage, resilience, and support. You know it, and now they know it, too!

* * *

CONCLUSION

Christian loosened his tie and slumped down in his chair. His colleague, Alana, perched on the chair opposite, grinning from ear to ear.

"Does it hurt?" she asked.

Christian gave her a puzzled look.

"You know, being on *fire*!" she added.

He chuckled. "Today was a good day," he agreed.

"Good?" she cried. "You were incredible! You must be the best spine surgeon in the whole country right now."

He shrugged self-consciously and looked away.

It was Alana's turn to look puzzled. "Why so shy?" she asked. "Surely you're used to praise; you must have been the smartest kid all through school and college."

"Well, actually..." He hesitated. "School was tough for me. I have ADHD, and for a while there, everyone thought I was headed nowhere."

"Jeez. What changed?"

"My parents," he said simply. "They believed in me. They never gave up. Because of their guidance, I was able to get myself together. They helped me to get organized and play to my strengths. I started high school as one of those kids they don't expect to graduate. And I finished with straight As. My success now is all thanks to the work they put in back then. I'll always be grateful."

***

As we reach the end of this book together, I want to take a moment to thank you for everything you have done and will continue to do for your ADHD teen. Any time that fear creeps back in and you wonder if there is hope for your kid, I want you to remember all the stories you have found here and all the skills you have learned.

There is so much more to ADHD than negativity. With your help and support, your teen can and will overcome their unique challenges. By implementing the strategies, activities, exercises, and tips you have learned, you can guide them toward success and a brighter future.

Now, it's time to put everything in this book into action. We began by learning all about ADHD and its traits, challenges, and treatments. Then, we dove deep into learning how to help your teen navigate the school environment with their diagnosis. We worked on organization, study styles, goal-setting, and other useful tools to help them with their learning. The final part of this book takes a close look at ADHD at home and in life in general. We discovered the emotional regulation mountains that your teen might struggle with, alongside their social skills and self-esteem.

Through it all, I hope that you have learned to trust yourself and your bond with your teen. There is nothing you can't overcome if you do it together. You can help them discover their strengths and utilize them, reframe their setbacks as lessons and opportunities, and emphasize their effort over perfection and achievement.

What's next? You decide. Your teenager is going to do beautiful things in the world; thank you for guiding them.

Activity 45: My Teen's Bright Future Journal Prompt

I have one final activity for you in this workbook. Looking back at everything we explored to help your teen manage their ADHD obstacles creatively across home, school, and life, take a moment to envision their path ahead thanks to the skills you have built together. You can use the journaling space provided to make notes:

What untapped strengths and passions now seem possible and will help them drive their future and thrive on their own terms?

How will understanding their differences, planning/ focus aids, and social courage change their future?

Describe your biggest hopes for who they are becoming and achieving, thinking about their unique interests years down the road. Consider what incredible careers they might have, what adventures abroad await them where they can connect to global communities, or perhaps artistic fame lies in their future, where they can showcase their talents through art.

THANK YOU

I would like to really thank you for reading my book till the end and, most importantly, applying as much as you can from what you learned here, as nothing would make me happier than knowing that someone's life is getting better because of something I shared!

I consider myself leveraged because you chose my book over all the other books to discover.

So, THANK YOU for purchasing this book and for making it all the way here.

Before you leave, I would like to ask for a favour! **Could you please share one or two things you learned or liked about this book in a review? That would really help me continue sharing more knowledge and would show your support to an independent author like myself!**

Your opinion will assist and encourage me to keep writing and publishing useful content for more people, hoping to make more people happier and enjoy their dream lives. Hearing from you would mean so much to me.

>> Leave a review on Amazon US <<

>> Leave a review on Amazon UK <<

REFERENCES

Seven ways to combat negative self-talk. (2018, May 4). Footprints to Recovery | Drug Rehab & Alcohol Addiction Treatment Centers. https://footprintstorecovery.com/blog/combat-negative-self-talk/

ADDA Editorial Team. (2023a, January 24). *Executive function disorder & ADHD.* Attention Deficit Disorder Association. https://add.org/executive-function-disorder/#:~:text=ADHD%20affects%20executive%20functioning%20%E2%80%93%20the

ADDA Editorial Team. (2023b, July 24). *Impact of ADHD at work.* Attention Deficit Disorder Association. https://add.org/impact-of-adhd-at-work/

ADDitude Editors. (2016a, November 28). *Famous people with ADHD.* ADDitude. https://www.additudemag.com/slideshows/famous-people-with-adhd/

ADDitude Editors. (2016b, November 29). *What I would never trade away.* ADDitude. https://www.additudemag.com/slideshows/positives-of-adhd/

ADHD in social situations | Attention deficit hyperactivity disorder. (n.d.). Adult ADHD Clinic. https://

adhdclinic.co.uk/adhd-in-social-situations/#:~:text=In%20social%20situations%2C%20the%20mood

American Academy of Pediatrics. (2019, September 27). *Common ADHD medications & treatments for children.* HealthyChildren. https://www.healthychildren.org/English/health-issues/conditions/adhd/Pages/Determining-ADHD-Medication-Treatments.aspx

Arguinchona, J. H., & Tadi, P. (2019, November 9). *Neuroanatomy, Reticular Activating System.* Nih.gov; StatPearls Publishing. https://www.ncbi.nlm.nih.gov/books/NBK549835/

Attention-Deficit / hyperactivity disorder (ADHD) in children. (n.d.). John Hopkins Medicine. https://www.hopkinsmedicine.org/health/conditions-and-diseases/adhdadd

Bailey, C. (n.d.). *Hyperfocus quotes.* Goodreads. https://www.goodreads.com/work/quotes/58759616-hyperfocus-how-to-be-more-productive-in-a-world-of-distraction#:~:text=by%20focusing%20deeply%20on%20just,most%20productive%20version%20of%20ourselves.

Ball, L. (n.d.). *Self acceptant quotes.* Goodreads. https://www.goodreads.com/quotes/tag/self-acceptance

Belsky, G. (2019, August 5). *What is executive function?* Understood. https://www.understood.org/articles/what-is-executive-function

Belsky, G. (n.d.). *Types of executive function skills.* Understood. https://www.understood.org/articles/

types-of-executive-function-skills

Brain-based techniques for retention of information. (2019). School of Medicine Loma Linda University. https://medicine.llu.edu/academics/resources/brain-based-techniques-retention-information

Breit, S., Kupferberg, A., Rogler, G., & Hasler, G. (2018). Vagus nerve as modulator of the brain–gut axis in psychiatric and inflammatory disorders. *Frontiers in Psychiatry, 9*(44). https://doi.org/10.3389/fpsyt.2018.00044

Brown, L. (n.d.). *Goals quotes.* BrainyQuote. https://www.brainyquote.com/quotes/les_brown_391112?src=t_goals

Burch, K. (2022, January 7). *What are benefits of having ADHD?* Verywell Health. https://www.verywellhealth.com/benefits-of-adhd-strengths-and-superpowers-5210520

Centers for Disease Control and Prevention. (2023, September 27). *What is ADHD?* https://www.cdc.gov/ncbddd/adhd/facts.html

Conway, W. E. (n.d.). *Top 40 productivity quotes.* QuoteFancy. https://quotefancy.com/productivity-quotes

Cuncic, A. (2022, November 9). *What is active listening?* Verywell Mind. https://www.verywellmind.com/what-is-active-listening-3024343

Data and statistics about ADHD. (2022, August 9). Centers for Disease Control and Prevention. https://www.cdc.gov/ncbddd/adhd/data.html

Davis, S. (n.d.). *The psychology behind why we love completing to-dos.* Workast. https://www.workast.com/blog/the-secret-psychology-on-why-we-love-completing-to-do-lists/#:~:text=When%20we%20complete%20individual%20tasks

Diamond, A. (2013). Executive functions. *Annual Review of Psychology, 64*(1), 135–168. https://doi.org/10.1146/annurev-psych-113011-143750

Ellis, R. R., & Seed, S. (2017, September 5). *What's the best exercise to manage ADHD symptoms?* WebMD. https://www.webmd.com/add-adhd/exercise-manage-adhd-symptoms

Everson, M. (2023, September 1). *Mindfulness by Miles: Here's why HANDWRITTEN notes are your ultimate weapon to supercharging your learning power....* LinkedIn. https://www.linkedin.com/pulse/mindfulness-miles-heres-why-handwritten-notes-your-ultimate-everson

Famous people with ADHD. (2022, August 12). ADHD UK. https://adhduk.co.uk/famous-people-with-adhd/

Fleming, G. (2018a). *Study strategies for the visual learning style.* ThoughtCo. https://www.thoughtco.com/visual-learning-style-p2-1857113

ABOUT THE AUTHOR

Kai M. Jordan

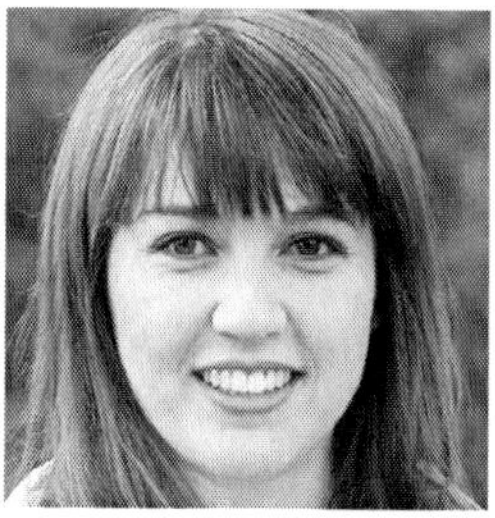

Kai M. Jordan is an author in the field of self-development, home management and lifestyle coach. Visit http://swenettbooks.com and get access to Kai's Decluttering Bundle for FREE.

In her books, Kai shares over ten years of practical knowledge and the timeless wisdom she learned from an early age about managing homes, mind and life by self-discovery, and self-management. She turns these life lessons into actionable steps to help you develop a healthy relationship with yourself, with others, and ultimately with life itself.

In her honest and inspiring books, Kai talks about what she believes are the obstacles to living the life you desire. She shares best practices to help you declutter your home, mind & life, improve powerful habits, erase negativity, control anxiety, reduce overthinking, and minimize any expectations of others. She guides YOU to think, decide and become the best version of yourself.

Kai studied business administration and project management. When she's not on her mission to make people's life better, she loves to read, meditate, workout, and take long walks in nature.

FOCUS FORWARD: NAVIGATING ADHD

Introducing the "Focus Forward: Navigating ADHD Series," a comprehensive guide designed to support individuals and families navigating the challenges of Attention Deficit Hyperactivity Disorder (ADHD). This transformative series comprises three essential volumes, each tailored to address specific aspects of life affected by ADHD.

Book 1: "Thrive with Adult ADHD for Women" - Dive into a journey of self-discovery and empowerment as this book offers invaluable insights and strategies tailored specifically for women navigating adulthood with ADHD. From embracing strengths to overcoming challenges, discover how to thrive in various aspects of life while harnessing the unique gifts of ADHD.

Book 2: "Organizing your Home and Life with ADHD" - Say goodbye to chaos and welcome organization into your home and daily routines with this practical guide. Packed with actionable tips and customizable systems, this book provides the tools needed to create order amidst the challenges of ADHD. From decluttering spaces to managing time effectively, reclaim control over your environment and enhance productivity.

Book 3: "Parenting Teens with ADHD" - Empower yourself with expert guidance on navigating the complexities of parenting teenagers with ADHD. This book offers proven strategies for fostering communication, building resilience, and navigating the unique challenges of adolescence. From academic support to fostering self-esteem, equip yourself with the knowledge and tools needed to guide your teen toward success.

Join the Focus Forward: Navigating ADHD Series and embark on a journey of growth, understanding, and empowerment as you navigate life with ADHD.

Thrive With Adult Adhd Workbook For Women

Learn How to overcome ADHD distractions and stay Organized, Master Your Relationships, Control your Emotions, and advance your career, and finances with 30 practical exercises NOW!

Studies show a greater number of cases diagnosed with ADHD in the young women population every year, pressure from society and women-related struggles play a factor in this.

Are you sick and tired of daily distractions and struggling to focus on one thing for some time?

Have you tried countless other focusing methods and techniques for ADHD but nothing seems to work?

Do you finally want to say goodbye to ADHD symptoms and discover something that actually works for you?

If so, then this book is for you.

Living a worry-free life from ADHD doesn't have to be complicated.

Even if you've tried other solutions that didn't work.

The truth is, it's much simpler than you think.

Amazon Best-selling author, Kai M. Jordan provides you with a step-by-step blueprint to overcome ADHD distractions and improve your focus, relationships, career, financials and all other aspects of your life without overwhelming yourself with complicated approaches and strategies.

In Thrive with Adult ADHD Workbook for Women, you'll discover:

* The biggest mistake people make when living and dealing with ADHD prevents them from enjoying a peaceful distraction-free life.

* The only techniques you need to know for a more successful, focused, and enjoyable life with ADHD.

* The 5 ways to live your dream life distraction-free with 30 practical exercises to apply throughout the year.

* Secrets to a happier, healthier and stress-free life

without sacrificing all your time and mental energy to achieve it.

* What Dr. Michele Novotni said about the relationship between Decluttering and ADHD!!

* Why your distraction level is hurting your progress – and what to do to overcome it.

* The best yearly plan with 30 exercises crafted carefully for you using scientifically proven strategies to help you on your journey to thrive with adult ADHD.

* Practical strategies, solutions, tips and tricks to control your relationships, deal with rejections, declutter your home, manage your relationships, manage your finances and improve your career.

...and so much more!

Imagine how you'll feel once you enjoy your life distraction-free, more relaxed and focused on your goals while controlling your ADHD, and how your life could change for the better.

So if you're currently suffering from ADHD symptoms, you can now rewire your brain, take back control of your stuff and enjoy a more peaceful life with Thrive with Adult ADHD Workbook for Women!

Organizing Your Home And Life With Adhd

Unlock the Secrets to a Tranquil Life: How to Conquer

Chaos and Thrive with ADHD!

Do you often find yourself drowning in clutter, battling distraction at every turn, and feeling like you're barely keeping it together?

Have you wished for a roadmap to navigate the challenges of home and life organization, specifically tailored for individuals with ADHD?

Imagine a life where chaos is replaced by calm, and each day is a step towards your goals. As someone who has walked in your shoes, I know the struggles, frustrations, and yearning for a system that truly works.

Are you tired of the endless cycle of disorganization, procrastination, and overwhelm?

What if you could transform your space into a haven of productivity and peace?

Picture a life where you can harness the unique strengths of your ADHD mind to create a home and lifestyle that supports your success. It's not a dream – it's a reality waiting for you.

Amazon best-selling author Kai M. Jordan, understands the daily battle with ADHD intimately. With a background in life coaching and years of experience working with individuals facing ADHD-related challenges, Jordan brings both professional expertise and personal understanding to this comprehensive guide. Having triumphed over organizational chaos personally, the author shares insights that go beyond generic advice.

* Discover practical strategies to declutter your physical space and clear mental fog.

* Unleash the power of ADHD-friendly routines that enhance focus and productivity.

* Learn the art of setting realistic and achievable goals tailored to your unique strengths.

* Navigate time management challenges with innovative techniques.

* Harness the potential of technology to streamline tasks and stay on track.

* Transform your living space into an organized sanctuary that supports your well-being.

* Dive into mindfulness practices designed to calm the chaos within.

* Equip yourself with coping mechanisms to overcome daily obstacles and thrive.

BOOKS BY THIS AUTHOR

Decluttering Your Home In A Year Or Less! Workbook

For everyone who's tired of looking at the mess in their living situation, have you ever thought, "wow, I really wish this clutter would all just go away?"
Well, now it can! Just keep reading...
Do you suffer from the clutter all over your home?

Do you often struggle every time you want to start to declutter and get your home tidy not

knowing how to start?

Do you have a hard time letting go of your sentimental items?

If you answered yes to any of the previous questions, then keep reading...

How to get rid of all the mess and clutter in your home and life and keep your home tidy without sacrificing a lot of time or having additional daily chores, even if you've tried everything and nothing worked for you.

Imagine yourself relaxing in your tidy, organized clean home after you got rid of all unwanted stuff. Imagine even having your home tidy forever with very minimal effort. Imagine your life without all the stress and overwhelming feeling of guilt for seeing your home in a mess all the time. Say goodbye to complicated plans or techniques to keep your home tidy, you will discover simple but very powerful ways to declutter your home easily.

In Decluttering Your Home in a year or less! Workbook, you will discover:

◆ The 1 hidden reason why your home is messy in the first place!

◆ The only 3 powerful techniques you need to know for decluttering and tidying up.

◆ More than 40 fun exercises that are specially crafted for you to guide you through your decluttering journey!

◆ More than 20 mental guidance and reflection spaces carefully placed through the workbook to help you discover yourself more by journaling and reaching your goals easily!

◆ Secrets to get your home and life de-cluttered without giving away all your time in return!

◆ Why using the standard systematic decluttering and

organizing methods is hurting your progress and what to do instead.

◆ Why your existing tidying up and decluttering techniques are an extra burden with no clear results (and what to do about it).

◆ How to easily create your personal tailored decluttering plan that matches your goals.

◆ How to prioritize your decluttering sequence of items in the best proven order.

◆ Surprising advice from Dale Carnegie on how to make your plan works!

◆ .... and so much more!

Amazon #1best-selling author and decluttering expert Kai M. Jordan is introducing the Decluttering Your Home in a year or less! Workbook, now you'll have a book telling you to get off your couch and just freaking do it yourself! We got inspirational quotes, we got a load of in-your-face, no-nonsense hard facts to throw at your sense of laziness! Time to face the freaking facts, you're living in a bird's nest! With this handy-dandy guide, you'll be asking yourself, "Was that really necessary?" and to that, we say, "YEAH IT WAS, BECAUSE YOU DESERVE TO LIVE IN A TIDY, COZY AND ORGANIZED HOME! "

Now, don your cleaning clothes, tie your hair back if you have long enough hair to do that, and buckle up. It's time to take out the trash and begin our interesting journey in

Decluttering Your Home in a year or less! Workbook.

Declutter Your Mind In A Year Or Less!

Learn How To Talk To Yourself To Reduce Stress, Eliminate Mental Clutter, Stop Worrying, And Control Your Inner Voice NOW!
Are you sick and tired of mental clutter, negative thoughts and bad inner voice?

Have you tried countless other solutions but nothing seems to work?

Do you finally want to say goodbye to stress, negative inner voice and mental clutter and discover something that actually works for you?

If so, then this book is for you.

You see, living worry-free life with decluttered mind doesn't have to be complicated/difficult.

Even if you've tried other solutions that didn't work.

The truth is, it's much simpler than you think.

Amazon Best-selling author, Kai M. Jordan provides you with a step-by-step blueprint to Declutter Your Mind and Life without overwhelming yourself with complicated approaches and strategies.

In Declutter Your Mind In A Year Or Less!, you'll discover:

◆The biggest mistake people make when talking to themselves that prevents them from living a stress-free and healthy decluttered life.

◆The only 3 techniques you need to know for a decluttered mind and life.

◆The 5 ways to live your dream life with a worry-free and decluttered mind in just 7 minutes a day.

◆The 4 things you should know about your inner voice and how to tame it.

◆Secrets to happier, healthier and stress-free life without sacrificing all your time and mental energy to achieve it.

◆What Henry Ford said about self-talk!

◆Why thinking about your future all the time is hurting your progress – and what to do instead.

◆The best yearly plan with more than 20 exercises crafted carefully for you to help you on your journey to Declutter Your Mind.

◆...and so much more!

Imagine how you'll feel once you live your life stress-free with no negative thoughts, controlling your inner voice and enjoying your decluttered mind, and how your life could change for the better.

So if you're currently suffering from the self-deprecating talk, having many more sleepless nights with racing thoughts, you can now rewire your brain and enjoy a more peaceful life with Declutter Your Mind In A Year Or Less!

Organize Your Digital Life

Learn How To Manage Your Social Media and Organize Your Digital world To Connect with Your Inner Self, Control Your Technology, Have More Fun, And re-Discover the Offline World NOW!
Are you sick and tired of digital clutter, increasing world distractions and overwhelming social media pressure?

Have you tried countless other solutions to take back control of your life but nothing seems to work?

Do you finally want to say goodbye to distractions, digital noise and overwhelming social media life and discover something that actually works for you?

If so, then this book is for you.

You see, living distraction-free with organized digital life and better "real" relationships doesn't have to be complicated/difficult.

Even if you've tried other solutions that didn't work.

The truth is, it's much simpler than you think.

Amazon Best-selling author, Kai M. Jordan provides you with a step-by-step blueprint and a 21-day plan to Organize Your Digital Life and apply a digital detox without overwhelming yourself with complicated approaches and strategies.

In Organize Your Digital Life, you'll discover:

✓ The biggest mistake people make when dealing with their digital life that prevents them from living a focused and healthy life in our noisy world.

✓ The only 3 steps plan you need to apply today for an organized digital life.

✓ The 5 ways to live your dream life with worry-free and organized technology in just 21 days.

✓ The 5 things you should know about the relationship between your mental and physical health.

✓ Secrets to happier, healthier and stress-free life without sacrificing all your time and mental energy to achieve it.

✓ What Mark Twain said about the detox concept!

✓ Why pushing the LIKE button on social media is hurting your progress – and what to do instead.

✓ The best 21-day plan with 6 powerful practical exercises crafted carefully for you using scientifically proven strategies to help you on your journey to control your digital world.

✓ ...and so much more!

Imagine how you'll feel once you live your life distraction-free with real healthy relationships, managing your social media and digital world effectively, and how your life could change for the better.

So if you're currently suffering from less productivity, low-quality relationships, digital distractions having many more sleepless nights with racing thoughts, you can now rewire your brain and enjoy a more peaceful life with Organize Your Digital Life.

Organize Your Home In A Year Or Less!

Learn How To Keep Your House Under Control, Bring any Home out of its mess, Master the Magic of Organization and Enjoy Being At Home NOW with 12 Practical Exercises!

Are you sick and tired of your messy home, disorganized rooms and things away from its place?

Have you tried countless other organization solutions but nothing seems to work?

Do you finally want to say goodbye to mess, overpacked kitchen cabinets, kids toys everywhere and discover something that actually works for you?

If so, then this book is for you.

You see, living a worry-free life with a beautiful organized home doesn't have to be complicated.

Even if you've tried other solutions that didn't work.

The truth is, it's much simpler than you think.

Amazon Best-selling author, Kai M. Jordan provides you with a step-by-step blueprint to Organize Your Home and Life without overwhelming yourself with complicated approaches and strategies.

In Organize Your Home In A Year Or Less!, you'll discover:

* The biggest mistake people make when Organizing their homes that prevents them from enjoying a peaceful life in an organized home, and how to understand Decluttering Vs Organizing.

* The only 3 techniques you need to know for an organized home and life.
The 5 ways to live your dream life with an organized home with 12 practical exercises to apply throughout the year.

* The 4 things you should know about the difference between Decluttering and Organizing.
Secrets to a happier, healthier and organized life without sacrificing all your time and mental energy to achieve it.

* What Benjamin Franklin said about Organizing!

* Why your stress level is hurting your progress – and

what to do to overcome it.

* The best yearly plan with 12 exercises crafted carefully for you using scientifically proven strategies to help you on your journey to organize your home.

* Practical strategies, solutions, tips and tricks to organize your kitchen, living area, bathroom, kids room, garage, attic, bedroom, closet, sentimental items, maintenance and cleaning.
...and so much more!

Imagine how you'll feel once you enjoy your life in your organized and clean homewhile controlling your stuff, and how your life could change for the better.

So if you're currently suffering from a messy and disorganized house, you can now rewire your brain, take back control of your stuff and enjoy a more peaceful life with Organize Your Home In A Year Or Less!

Made in United States
North Haven, CT
10 November 2026

22096037R00129